Critical Thinking and Writing in Nursing

6E

Bob Price

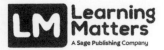

Learning Matters
A Sage Publishing Company
1 Oliver's Yard
55 City Road
London EC1Y 1SP

Sage Publications Inc.
2455 Teller Road
Thousand Oaks, California 91320

Sage Publications India Pvt Ltd
B 1/I 1 Mohan Cooperative Industrial Area
Mathura Road
New Delhi 110 044

Sage Publications Asia-Pacific Pte Ltd
3 Church Street
#10-04 Samsung Hub
Singapore 049483

Editor: Martha Cunneen
Development editor: Sarah Turpie
Senior project editor: Chris Marke
Project management: Westchester Publishing
Services UK
Marketing manager: Ruslana Khatagova
Cover design: Sheila Tong
Typeset by: C&M Digitals (P) Ltd, Chennai, India
Printed and bound by CPI Group (UK) Ltd,
Croydon, CR0 4YY

Library of Congress Control Number: 2023944521

British Library Cataloguing in Publication data

A catalogue record for this book is available from the
British Library

ISBN 978-1-5296-6660-1
ISBN 978-1-5296-6659-5 (pbk)

At Sage we take sustainability seriously. Most of our products are printed in the UK using responsibly sourced
papers and boards. When we print overseas we ensure sustainable papers are used as measured by the Paper
Chain Project grading system. We undertake an annual audit to monitor our sustainability.

Contents

TRANSFORMING NURSING PRACTICE

Transforming Nursing Practice is a series tailor made for pre-registration student nurses. Each book in the series is:

✓ Affordable

✓ Full of active learning features

✓ Mapped to the NMC Standards of proficiency for registered nurses

✓ Focused on applying theory to practice

Each book addresses a core topic and they have been carefully developed to be simple to use, quick to read and written in clear language.

An invaluable series of books that explicitly relates to the NMC standards. Each book covers a different topic that students need to explore in order to develop into a qualified nurse... I would recommend this series to all Pre-Registered nursing students whatever their field or year of study.

LINDA ROBSON,
Senior Lecturer at Edge Hill University

Many titles in the series are on our recommended reading list and for good reason - the content is up to date and easy to read. These are the books that actually get used beyond training and into your nursing career.

EMMA LYDON,
Adult Student Nursing

ABOUT THE SERIES EDITORS

DR MOOI STANDING is an Independent Nursing Consultant (UK and International) and is responsible for the core knowledge, adult nursing and personal and professional learning skills titles. She is an experienced NMC Quality Assurance Reviewer of educational programmes and a Professional Regulator Panellist on the NMC Practice Committee. Mooi is also Board member of Special Olympics Malaysia, enabling people with intellectual disabilities to participate in sports and athletics nationally and internationally.

DR SANDRA WALKER is a Clinical Academic in Mental Health working between Southern Health Trust and the University of Southampton and responsible for the mental health nursing titles. She is a Qualified Mental Health Nurse with a wide range of clinical experience spanning more than 25 years.

BESTSELLING TEXTBOOKS

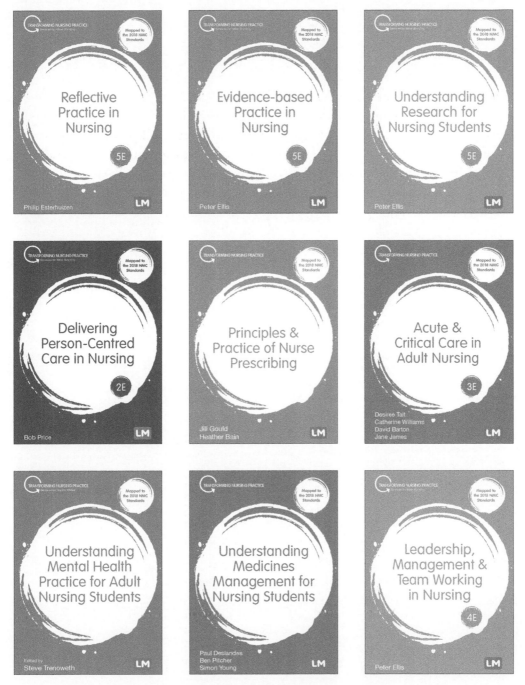

You can find a full list of textbooks in the *Transforming Nursing Practice* series at

https://uk.sagepub.com/TNP-series

About the author

Bob Price is a healthcare education and training consultant. Formerly, he was Director, Postgraduate Awards in Advancing Healthcare Practice at the Open University. A passionate educator, he has assisted students at every level, from pre-registration programmes of study up to and including PhD. Bob's doctoral thesis was on the negotiation of learning and ways to assist students with their studies. He is an editorial adviser to a range of healthcare journals, advising editors on teaching texts and student learning needs.

Acknowledgements

This book would not have been possible, without the case study nurse contributions of Stewart, Fatima, Raymet, Gina and Sue, who very generously agreed to explore critical thinking and reflection with me through their own studies. The book certainly would not have made it to the printed and e-learning pages without the support and very constructive feedback of critical readers, Series Editor Dr Mooi Standing, Martha Cunneen (Commissioning Editor) and the rest of the editorial team at Sage.

Foreword

Critical Thinking and Writing in Nursing facilitates the development of essential personal and professional learning skills by carefully guiding readers in how to process information and then articulate and apply what they have learned. Readers' personal development is facilitated in acquiring, understanding and demonstrating critical thinking, reflecting and scholarly writing skills. This goes hand in hand with facilitating their professional development in the wide variety of learning situations that they experience, and in nurturing and applying critical thinking skills in their formal academic and practical assessments. Readers are encouraged to engage with lots of interesting and challenging activities that combine and progressively stretch their personal and professional learning skills in reflecting and thinking critically. Case studies chart the progress of four pre-registration nursing students to illustrate different perspectives and learning styles in acquiring and applying critical thinking skills in providing a high standard of nursing care for patients. In this way the book succeeds in preparing nursing students for the challenges faced by registered nurses including demonstrating critical thinking and reflection to satisfy revalidation requirements.

The author has updated and revised the sixth edition of this highly regarded book to further reduce the theory-practice gap by showing how skilled nursing practice incorporates critical thinking within person-centred care. In doing so Bob Price succeeds in making a complex topic more accessible, understandable and applicable for nurses to evaluate and enhance their care of patients. I can therefore wholeheartedly recommend this excellent book to all nursing students, registered nurses, practice supervisors/assessors and nurse educators.

Dr Mooi Standing

Series Editor

Introduction

The ability to think critically, to reflect upon experience and then to write about such matters in a clear fashion is central to your success, both while studying a programme of nursing studies and later when demonstrating your readiness to revalidate as a registered nurse (NMC, 2019). *The Code* (NMC, 2018a) requires nurses to attend safely, sensitively, effectively, imaginatively and efficiently to patient care, and this is underpinned by both critical thinking and reflection. Together, critical thinking and reflecting shape what it means to learn at university. You will be completing your studies at a pivotal time, one where new technology is shaping how subjects are taught and developing what you are expected to master through personal enquiry. While historically we have thought of study as attending lectures and using the library, you will discover that university mixes and matches your learning opportunities in new ways that will help you to become a confident lifelong learner. This book is designed to assist you with this process.

The book has a further purpose, however – one that is very personal. This relates to helping you to think in ways that help you to endure within nursing. Healthcare practice is full of challenges. While we work within a code of practice and with clinical guidelines and protocols, there are still different ways to care for patients. There are often difficulties in negotiating the right care with patients and their families. There are equally challenges associated with allocating scant resources and prioritising care when demands compete for your time. While much is taught to you, and much is recommended, you will still have to deliberate on what is practicable, ethical and professional. What is acceptable to the patient (informed consent), what is recommended as ideal (professional philosophy) and what is practicable (health service economics) are not always the same. Addressing the many competing demands about what you should do is stressful. For that reason, this book is also about judging the practical utility of information, theories and arguments. Success sometimes depends upon the skill you have in navigating the practical as well as the desirable.

Who is this book for?

This book has been written for two audiences: students completing nursing courses (basic and post-basic levels) and registered nurses who are charged with demonstrating their continued learning and enquiry as part of the revalidation process (NMC, 2019). While the requirements of critical thinking and reflection may vary (e.g. associated with the level of course studied), the processes remain much the same. The nurse must process that which is discovered, interpreting and sorting it before care decisions can be made.

Because the book starts with the basics, it is designed to reassure and support those of you who may not have studied for some time. I begin with the assumption that critical thinking, reflecting and writing are three of the craft skills of nursing.

Much of what is best in nursing is defined by the way in which we deliver care as much as by what is provided. For this reason, reading this book will start you on a journey where you discover how best to use your experience in the service of others. This is a process that draws heavily upon making sense of practice, exploring what you believe is best within nursing care, and planning future development that helps you to express your thinking more effectively.

Critical thinking and reflecting

One of the earliest discoveries made by student nurses is how often the word 'critical' appears in their work. In the clinical context, the word carries connotations of risk and the need for urgent intervention (e.g. 'a patient is critically ill') (Kayambankzanya et al., 2022). Used in this sense, the nurse quickly realises the need for precision and judgement, the requirement to do the right thing, in the right way and at the right time. In the academic context, 'critical' takes on several different meanings (Merisier et al., 2018). You are asked to 'critically discuss', 'critically evaluate' and 'critically explore' a subject, and it slowly becomes apparent that to be critical involves different things, depending on the teaching or assessment involved. For example, to be critical in this context might mean to discriminate between what is right and wrong, defensible and indefensible. Asking the right questions of information or a clinical situation is important. If you are preparing a reflective piece of writing, then 'critical' often involves being introspective, examining afresh your beliefs, values and motives.

In this book, I use the term 'critical thinking' in a particular way. It describes the process by which we develop powers of analysis and investigation, as well as enhancing our ability to discriminate what is relevant and to discern what might prove most helpful. Critical thinking may have to work in situations where there is no absolute truth, no perfect answers, only better ones. Much as we might yearn for certainty, there are times in healthcare when none can be promised.

Critical thinking involves judgement, and nurses are frequently assessed on their decision-making skills (Clemett and Raleigh, 2021). A competent nurse is one who selects the relevant information to plan a course of action and then judges what is best to do in a given circumstance (Casey et al., 2017). We are best placed to improve care where we have the capacity to reason what is not yet understood and what will enable us to be more imaginative, sensitive, respectful, and efficient and effective in what we do.

While 'critical' is sometimes encountered in a more destructive form within practice (e.g. where practitioners belittle others' shortfalls), this is not the sense in which we will use it here. Indeed, I suggest that the individual who criticises without consideration of what is learned through the experience is demonstrating neither scholarship nor professionalism.

It is likely that you have already engaged in reflection as part of previous studies. For example, at school, you perhaps judged which subjects to take to examination based on your past comfort with them in class. However, in nursing, reflection has a very important and specific role. It is strongly associated with the development of empathy (i.e. the understanding of and respect for the circumstances of others) (Jack and Levatt-Jones, 2022). Nurses need to be emotionally intelligent, anticipating how illness, treatment and care might seem to patients and how different courses of action might seem to professional colleagues. Without adequate empathy, there is a significant risk that patients may be neglected. Because nurses are asked to use their experience and their insights as part of nursing care, reflection takes on a special meaning. While at least some of your teaching in college starts with concepts or theories that describe the world of healthcare, much of what you learn through practice starts from episodes of care that are much more ambiguous. We must make sense of what is going on. Evidence alone will not secure the healthcare improvements that we strive for. Not surprisingly, then, both critical thinking and reflection are important. Critical thinking engages our reasoning as we ponder theories, evidence, arguments and debates, while reflection does the same as we contemplate experience.

How this book is set out

This book is set out in three parts. You will dip in again later. Part 1 consists of three chapters that introduce you in an accessible way to the key concepts which feature in this book: critical thinking, reflecting and scholarly writing. Securing a basic idea about what these are all about will help you to make a great deal more sense of what is asked of you upon a course. Within Part 1, I introduce you to different levels of critical thinking and reflection, something that you will need to understand in order to understand tutor feedback and pass module assessments.

Part 2 concerns the use of reasoning and reflection within different contexts. It will help you to understand what is involved in getting the most from a variety of learning opportunities, including lectures, demonstrations, seminars, workshops and clinical placements. Much of what I write about here relating to learning in university contexts applies equally well to the registered nurse preparing for revalidation. Conferences and study days, for example, are often arranged as a series of lectures and smaller 'breakout' group discussions.

On your course, you are asked to engage in different learning activities for a reason, and this includes building confidence in your own enquiries. It is not the teacher's objective to drill you in a set way of thinking. Rather, they hope to acquaint you with different approaches to enquiry and understanding. Sometimes teaching precedes a programme of library enquiry. You are assisted in deciding, for example, whether a theory holds good in all circumstances (deductive learning). Sometimes you are tasked with personal enquiries in order to build a theory of your own (inductive learning). The organisation of studies within a module will have a specific purpose, although that might not always be apparent! Your course is likely to require very active learning; it will not be sufficient to sit, wait and take notes.

If Part 2 is about the process of learning then Part 3 is about the process of expressing what you have learned. This part opens with a chapter on evaluating evidence. During your nursing career, you will have access to a wide range of evidence of varying quality, so it is vital that you can reason to best effect. I assist you with the matter of writing different sorts of essays (analytical and reflective) and building a portfolio that helps you to demonstrate your progress. While there are many forms that assessment can take in nursing courses, the principles of analytical and reflective writing remain firm. In this part, we spend some time illustrating how you can demonstrate the different levels of critical thinking that may be required at different stages of your course. Part 3 also includes a new chapter on writing clinical case studies, something that will be important when justifying the planning of patient support over a series of care episodes. The clinical case study helps you to link reflective practice skills and critical analysis of evidence together.

Learning features

Throughout the book, you will find activities that will help you to make sense of and learn about the material presented.

Some of the activities ask you to *reflect* on aspects of practice. Other activities ask you to *think critically* about a topic in order to challenge received wisdom. You may be asked to *research a topic and find appropriate information and evidence*, as well as to be able to *make decisions* using that evidence.

All of the activities require you to take a break from reading the text, think through the issues presented, and carry out some independent study, possibly using the internet. You might want to think about completing the activities as part of your portfolio.

NMC Future Nurse: Standards of Proficiency for Registered Nurses

In 2018, the UK's NMC published its Future Nurse: Standards of Proficiency for Registered Nurses (NMC, 2018b), describing what registered nurses must be able to demonstrate at the conclusion of their nurse education. Relevant standards are detailed at the start of each chapter in this book.

Supporting the NMC code of professional practice

In addition to the above standards, this book works closely with the NMC code of professional practice (*The Code*).

The Code (NMC, 2018a) describes four areas of professional responsibility:

- prioritise people;
- practise effectively;
- preserve safety;
- promote professionalism and trust.

Prioritise people

Nurses are required to attend quickly, considerately, respectfully and compassionately to other people, both the service users within healthcare and their colleagues in practice. Nurses must be able to analyse others' likely needs and concerns, as well as respecting their confidentiality and individuality while doing so. It is important for nurses to listen to the experience of patients and what they relate about their expectations of care.

Practise effectively

It is not enough that nurses are respectful and considerate towards patients; they must be effective as well. Healthcare resources, be they medicines, materials or the nurse's time, are scarce resources and must be used to best effect. To work effectively, *The Code* requires that nurses make the best possible use of evidence, communicate clearly, work co-operatively and share their skills and expertise with others.

Critical thinking (Chapter 1) is important in efficient and effective practice. What will work best, and why? What is the best order in which to do things? Why might it be better to act in one way than another? Chapter 8 helps you to better understand evidence that stems from research, clinical audit and clinical case studies. Although evidence may recommend a particular course of action, it may not seem the best or most desirable course of action to the patient, so reflection (Chapter 2) is important here as well. A nurse might need to 'sell' the benefits of a recommended course of action to a patient.

Preserve safety

Nurses have the potential to cause considerable harm and to do great good. With this in mind, *The Code* requires that nurses work within the limits of their competence, as well as within the protocols and policies established by healthcare organisations. They must be prepared to raise concerns where patients seem at risk and to intervene in emergencies where they have the requisite competence to do so. Nurses must be prepared to acknowledge mistakes or errors, as well as act quickly and collaboratively to mitigate these where possible.

Judging exactly what you know, as well as how confident this might make you feel, is important. What you read about in Chapter 1 (critical thinking) and Chapter 2 (reflection), as well as what you learn in Chapter 3 (scholarly writing), will prompt you to examine again what supports your decision-making. Safety often relies upon judging when not to act, when it is better to consult or refer, and this in turn relies upon a willingness to examine why something seems like a good idea.

Promote professionalism and trust

The Code reminds nurses of their professional responsibility to uphold the reputation of the profession, as well as their own status as a nurse. To this end, they must act without favour and not accept loans or gifts that might otherwise influence their professional judgement or the reputation of the profession. They must respond promptly and considerately to complaints, as well as exercising leadership as part of their work to promote the well-being of patients and excellence in care standards. Registered nurses are expected to carry on learning, refining and improving their professional skills, and mastering new knowledge or approaches to care that reflect what evidence has taught.

Being ready to examine complaints honestly, as well as confronting suspect practice, relies upon our readiness to judge evidence and explain our reasoning. What is excellent? What is suspect? What could lead to harm or difficulty for the patient? We will need to think objectively and critically (Chapter 1), as well as reflecting on events, even though this causes us to revisit our own values and beliefs (Chapter 2).

Part 1   Understanding thinking, reflecting and writing

Chapter 1 Critical thinking

NMC Future Nurse: Standards of Proficiency for Registered Nurses

This chapter will address the following platforms and proficiencies:

Platform 1: Being an accountable professional

At the point of registration, the registered nurse will be able to:

1.8 Demonstrate the knowledge, skills and ability to think critically when applying evidence and drawing on experience to make evidence informed decisions in all situations.

1.9 Understand the need to base all decisions regarding care and interventions on people's needs and preferences, recognising and addressing any personal and external factors that may unduly influence their decisions.

1.18 Demonstrate the knowledge and confidence to contribute effectively and proactively in an interdisciplinary team.

Platform 3: Assessing needs and planning care

At the point of registration, the registered nurse will be able to:

3.5 Demonstrate the ability to accurately process all information gathered during the assessment process to identify needs for individualised nursing care and develop person-centred evidence-based plans for nursing interventions with agreed goals.

3.7 Understand and apply the principles and processes for making reasonable adjustments.

Chapter aims

After reading this chapter, you will be able to:

- define critical thinking in your own practical terms;
- discuss why this skill is important in nursing;
- summarise different aptitudes associated with critical thinking;
- indicate your level of confidence associated with each of the aptitudes of critical thinking;
- describe what constitutes more sophisticated forms of critical thinking.

Introduction

Let me start by setting a context for our discussion of critical thinking. Your career in nursing has never been more dependent upon the ability to reason effectively. Critical thinking is important for your personal well-being and your sense of progress. Here are three issues that highlight this:

1. The knowledge that we use to nurse today is much more complex, and it includes a mass of sometimes contradictory, incomplete or contentious information (Huber et al., 2021). This has implications when patients ask you for advice, and when they evaluate what you do. If we do not know how to evaluate complex information, to conceive of problems and solutions to best effect, then we will struggle to be successful carers.

2. Our knowledge operates where there remains a gulf between what could be done and what philosophers believe should be done (Salifu et al., 2019). Just as the demands of health consumers have increased, so have the aspirations of nursing as a profession. We hope to offer more bespoke care. What could and should be done, however, often conflict. You must work in settings where resources are finite. You cannot promise to deliver everything that everyone desires, so you must make difficult decisions about what you can offer. Those decisions involve the strategic use of information. This prompts a new question: Can I make these ideas work?

3. Nursing knowledge operates within the context of shifting roles and responsibilities (e.g. Boyne et al., 2022). What we do today is very different to what nurses did 20 years ago. In many areas, practice is extended, and nurses do work doctors did previously. Once upon a time, nurses talked about 'basic nursing care', but today we might struggle to agree what 'basic' means.

Activity 1.1   Reflection

Pause now to consider what such complex information and a changing context might mean for how you learn about nursing at university. For example, is absorbing material via lectures the most effective way to learn? Why might it be advantageous for you to learn how to explore problems or needs with others, and to conduct enquiries actively, in other settings such as the library?

My brief answer to such questions is given at the end of this chapter.

Critical thinking

We have been involved in reasoning throughout our lives. However, many of the past decisions that we have made have been managed without great analysis. We have behaved instinctively and accepted what seems 'common sense'. To be successful nurses, though, we need to practise the skill of critical thinking in a more conscious manner (Standing, 2020).

Critical thinking can be described as having two foci. The first entails the careful scrutiny of phenomena, processes, causes and effects. These are **empirical** things, facts, statistics, tests and results. This involves the exercise of what has been called **cognitive intelligence** (Barbey et al., 2021). When you assess a wound, for example, you examine the extent and depth of the wound, whether it is infected. The assessment is dispassionate and measured. But in nursing, critical thinking also involves an understanding of how we and others feel (e.g. what it involves to be ill). This is **emotional intelligence** (Tiffin and Paton, 2020). Nurses need to exercise emotional intelligence to deliver care well. If we don't understand what a patient believes and how they feel, we are less likely to build a rapport with them.

What, then, do we mean by critical thinking? I suggest that critical thinking is:

> *A process where different information is gathered, sifted, synthesised and evaluated in order to understand a subject or issue. Critical thinking engages our intellect (the ability to discriminate, challenge and argue), but it might engage our emotions too. To think critically, we need to take account of values, beliefs and attitudes that shape our perceptions. Critical thinking, then, is that which enables the nurse to function as a knowledgeable practitioner – someone who selects, combines, judges and uses information in order to proceed in a professional manner.*

Critical thinking and learning

To help you explore further, meet now four student nurses and one staff nurse who are helping us in this book. Stewart, Fatima, Raymet and Gina are students, while Sue is a staff nurse on a busy hospital ward. Sue's interest is in the use of critical thinking to prepare for revalidation (NMC, 2019), but she remembers what study was like. We will return to our case study nurses periodically throughout the book.

Our case study nurses meet up to discuss some of the challenges of completing a nursing course. While their studies are interesting, they all acknowledge that learning can be difficult because of the critical thinking required.

Activity 1.2   Reflection

Look now at the accounts in the box below of critical thinking challenges reported by our group.

* Have you encountered similar concerns?
* Why do you think that the case study nurse accounts tell us about how nurses have to think?

As this answer is based on your own observation, there is no outline answer at the end of the chapter.

Case study: Five critical thinking challenges

Stewart:	'I've realised not only that there is important theory to grasp, but that it isn't always simple to use in practice. Not everything in theory seems open to use. Some of it must be adjusted before you can use it. Maybe some of it is just nice to know?'
Fatima:	'For me, it's the uncertainty. I long for a right answer, something that I know is just correct, and a lot of what we're learning about – for instance, ethics – isn't so clear-cut.'
Raymet:	'I agree. But have you noticed just how much information there is? It's like they fill up your kitbag with everything you could ever want and then leave you to decide when to pull it out. The sheer volume is worrying.'
Gina:	'I wouldn't disagree with any of those points. But have you noticed how important it is to understand processes as well as purposes? You quickly learn what you should do, but how to do it is something more complex. It's that which I find myself admiring nurses for.'
Sue (registered nurse):	'Goodness, I remember those anxieties. The learning I do now for professional update is less structured. I must decide what I wish to improve upon, and then to judge the best ways to meet my needs. That means sometimes confronting care that I didn't get right. It means being candid with myself about the need to change what I do.'

You might already empathise with these five colleagues, each of whom describes something about critical thinking in nursing. Nursing practice relies heavily on the skills of the nurse, and central among these is the ability to reason. Skills are made up of a series of component parts, and it is the way in which these are combined and used that determines how skilful the practice seems (Gobet, 2005; Gobet and Chassy, 2008; Sala and Gobet, 2017) (see Figure 1.1). While the circumstances under which critical thinking must be exercised may change (e.g. an emergency versus palliative care), expert practitioners are still able to combine the components of critical thinking in ways which serve well (Sala and Gobet, 2017). This is because the ways of thinking in different situations (templates) are repeatedly tested by the nurse.

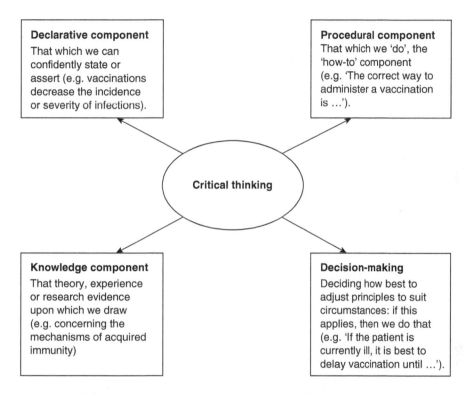

Figure 1.1　Critical thinking components of nursing skill

In the case study above, Stewart refers to the first of these components. Stewart worries about the application of theory. If we are going to deliver good nursing care, we must know how to combine and apply information. But information does not fit everywhere. So, for example, a series of seminars on grief might have value with dying patients, but wider application may be limited (it has limited **utility**). Not all information gleaned can be immediately used, nor is it universally taught for use in practice. Sometimes we learn things to appreciate how nursing has evolved. That said, however, we are usually faced with a challenge. We must be able to declare certain things (as true, sound, proven and/or relevant) if we are to build the confidence to care. Without that, we feel paralysed. What we need, then, is knowledge that has a frequent fit with clinical demands. It is not unreasonable to discuss the best fit use of information with your tutor. How abstract is the theory? Does it recognise the differences between patients, their histories and cultural backgrounds, for example?

Activity 1.3   Reflection

Try now to think of something within nursing that you must be able to assert confidently which also has utility (i.e. it is workable) in your chosen area of recent practice.

An outline answer is given at the end of this chapter.

Fatima refers to a second important component of critical thinking: *decision-making*. There is often no 'one-size-fits-all' solution. Fatima is keenly aware that nurses must deal with uncertainty, sometimes waiting to gather more information before deciding. Living with such uncertainty, especially in clinical practice, is what can seem stressful for nurses. They must learn to read developing situations and weigh the merits of different courses of action.

Raymet is worried about how best to artfully select and combine information to make excellent decisions. Established nurses seem to do it easily, explaining that they use 'nous'. The practice supervisors Raymet has met describe nous as a mix of thinking, remembering (from **experience**) and interpreting (how patients and relatives respond). We can only reason effectively if we have amassed enough high-quality knowledge that makes sense in the context of care (Ellis, 2019). Nurses must speculate how different bits of information might fit together to imagine how care could work. They must use both cognitive and emotional intelligence.

Activity 1.4   Reflection

Identify now one example of a difficult decision that you know about from clinical practice, or one that was debated in class. Was the decision of the either/or kind or was it more complicated, with multiple options and the merit of each dependent on factors such as patient preference?

An outline answer is given at the end of this chapter.

Both Gina and Sue refer to the *process* part of the skill. Reasoning is not only concerned with deciding what knowledge is appropriate, determining what is true, safe or effective, and making judicious decisions; it is also concerned with how you plan your work. When a nurse gives an injection, they determine the right order in which to proceed. The nurse first consults the patient about the planned injection, secures consent, and then ensures a private environment to help to protect the patient's dignity. Planning the right sequence of work is important, whether completing a clinical procedure or planning update enquiries.

Activity 1.5   Critical Thinking

Explore now with a chosen colleague an activity from your recent learning to determine the different ways in which reasoning has had to work (deciding what you can claim, making decisions, reviewing knowledge and deciding on process). Next compare notes with your colleague on which of the skill components seemed toughest, and why.

Because this activity focuses on your chosen learning activity, no additional remarks are added at the end of the chapter.

In my experience, it is often the **declarative critical thinking** component of a skill that seems hardest to students. There is sometimes no single 'right' answer, but there are better answers. To ascertain those, discussion and consultation with others is so important. That is why nursing courses build in so much discussion time and why you are asked to 'think aloud'. Qualified nurses confront the declarative skills component problem by conferring with colleagues and sometimes collaborating on case conferences. It is professionally important that nurses acknowledge what they are unsure about and are candid about any dilemmas that they face (NMC, 2018a).

No matter what part of the course you are studying, you will be engaged in critical thinking, combining and recombining the different components of nursing skills so that you can proceed in ways which seem professional. Nursing practice must be reasoned, and the actions of the nurse reasonable. Indeed, in a court of law, judgements about whether a nurse's actions are negligent are based upon what a reasonable practitioner would deduce or do (Baylis, 2015). What the case study nurses will learn throughout their course is designed to enable them to work more safely, strategically, effectively (achieving required outcomes) and efficiently (using resources wisely).

Building templates

You might wonder, what next? Once we appreciate that critical thinking involves these different skill components, what follows on from that? The brief answer is that you start to develop some **templates** to make better sense of what you have discovered, what you have been taught, and what you might then do. For templates to work you need to draw on relevant constituent concepts. A list of concepts that nurses regularly use might include pain, recovery, rehabilitation, support and effective listening. When the concepts combine to facilitate practical actions, responses to needs or concerns, we call them templates. 'Template' sounds like a technical term, but it simply means a working explanation of what we encounter and how we can best respond. Human beings develop templates from childhood (Gold et al., 2016). For example, babies learn very quickly to make distinctions between what is threatening and what is comforting. A smile represents friendliness, and a glare represents threat. As you get older, you develop strategies to respond to friendliness and threat – you have been building templates for a good many years.

In nursing, though, the building of templates should be rather more conscious. Much of your teaching is designed to help you to do that. The very best practice supervisors explain how they assess practice situations – they share their working templates. I asked Sue to help with this using an example of a template that she uses nearly every day of her working life. She chose allaying anxiety. Patients frequently exhibit anxiety, and the nurse needs a working template to deal with it. Here is what she said:

> *Anxiety is something you recognise as a pattern. Certain things go together again and again, and that enables you to predict what might cause anxiety and how it will emerge. When you anticipate it well and move to reassure the patient, they appreciate your care. So, for anxiety, the pattern includes things like sudden change, a lack of or too much information, words and terms that seem very technical, and doubts about their ability to control what happens next. That is what evokes anxiety. You counter anxiety using different tools – reassurance, yes, but giving patients room to express their fears as well. So, if you keep checking your solutions against anxiety, you develop a working template. It's something you can use while staying ready to think again if something new pops up.*

Your course is designed to help you to develop working templates that will help you to practise nursing. That is why you are taught theory, why you share seminars (exploring what works well together), and why it is good to ask practice supervisors about how they read clinical situations. When we think critically, we hope to recognise patterns of information, those that represent something important to us (e.g. risk, rehabilitation, relapse, cancer, depression, compassion).

To build these templates, though, we are going to have to engage in some important work that connects reasoning to study.

Making critical thinking work for you

I asked the case study nurses to tell me what seemed to count as critical thinking in their nursing course, what seemed to be especially valued. I wanted to know what they thought was welcomed by tutors. What they told me is shown in Table 1.1.

Student	Aptitude	The student said ...
Stewart	Asking questions	'If you don't ask questions, then you simply accept others' explanations, and that could be wrong. You must be inquisitive.'
Fatima	Discriminating	'I find that you need to show how you reach conclusions, weighing up information. You must show that you've thought about what is relevant.'
Raymet	Making arguments	'I don't think you can just hide behind what others have claimed. You must explain what you think and take a considered stance.'
Gina	Interpreting and speculating	'I think that you show why you think something is significant, so you explain why you focus on it. But it is also important to say when you are speculating what could be the case. Don't be arrogant.'

Table 1.1　Critical thinking aptitudes

Asking questions

Asking questions is certainly important, but individuals vary in their levels of confidence. Perhaps you worry that asking questions betrays an uncomfortable level of ignorance. Asking questions, though, especially when working with professional colleagues, is at the heart of healthcare. Questions are frequently used to clarify the best care options, and at best these involve patients being involved in decisions. Sometimes a seemingly naive question is the one that transforms everyone's understanding of a clinical situation. You may hear practice supervisors rehearsing questions aloud as an aid to planning care: 'If I want to teach Mrs Jones about her insulin therapy, what does she need to understand in order to keep her safe and help her to master injection-giving?'

You can improve your question-asking by:

- deciding exactly what you need to know – this will help you to be precise as regards what you ask about;
- formulating your question in a way that establishes your focus of interest – it is better, for instance, to link a question about patient experience to a contextual concern, such as preoperative anxiety;
- jotting down your question before you ask it – this will help you to explain what you wish to understand.

Discriminating

There comes a stage where we must discriminate between what is relevant and what is irrelevant, as well as what is true and what is false. Discrimination involves weighing up information and determining what seems sound and is supported by others. One example of discrimination in action is where a nurse searches for evidence to support a given practice. The nurse reasons that the information supplied through well-designed research studies is better than that derived from anecdotal evidence. If you are judging the claims made by others, one way of showing discrimination is to ponder the circumstances or conditions under which that claim might be false. 'Under what conditions might it be unsafe for the patient to remain at home to receive care?' is an example of a question that might be used.

A part of discrimination involves judging what can work in practice. Is theory always operable? Person-centred care, for example, is a theory that has significant appeal for nurses (me included), but it does make significant demands on patients as partners. The extent that we can demonstrate it may depend on the patient's readiness to collaborate, as well as the nurse's skill (Price, 2022).

Showing appropriate discrimination in your reasoning will be important in your written work. You will need to demonstrate that you have considered possible explanations of what you have read, as well as determining what you need to consider before you elect a particular course of action. In Part 3, we discuss different levels of critical thinking in your writing, and one of the markers of higher-level critical thinking is that not only can you identify what must be discriminated between (the competing explanations), but you can also reason why one explanation seems better than another. Where writing shows little or no recognition of competing explanations, it might be described as uncritical or even opinionated.

Making arguments

Arguments are formulated about a variety of things: what should be done next, what this literature suggests, and what constitutes compassionate care. Arguments are necessary, as they explain the basis of nursing in action and why we are working to the goals that we have. An argument is made up of a case (what we believe is true) and **premises** (the things that support the case) (Chatfield, 2022). Both the case and the premises may be supported by research evidence, audit and experience. So, for example, we might make an argument about patient anxiety and how it interferes with collaborative care planning: 'Collaborative care planning is made more difficult with anxious patients (the case) because patients have a limited command of relevant information, and they feel less powerful than clinicians (two supporting premises).' Notice the importance of the word 'because'. If we do not include what follows the case, we only present an opinion. We can only evaluate the argument if we understand on what basis the case is presented.

Classically, an argument such as this is judged regarding whether the premises and the case fit well together. Are the premises sufficient to support the case? But we might also consider whether the argument seems complete. There may be other factors that affect collaborative care planning (e.g. clinicians' willingness to consult with patients).

In nursing, the rationale for an argument may be based on evidence, but it might also be based on **moral justice** (Supady et al., 2021). Some arguments are made on ethical grounds regarding what *should* be done. A good way to strengthen your arguments within a debate is to show that you have carefully considered alternative arguments, namely other ways to see the situation. You then reject some arguments by offering a rationale for why they are weak (the premises do not support the case).

Activity 1.6   Collaborative practice

Have a go now formulating an argument for your colleagues to interrogate. Remember that the argument needs a case (that which you claim) and premises that support it. Typically, the case is presented first, and then after 'because' come the underpinning premises. Did your colleagues support your argument? If it seemed weak, what do you think the problem was? An unclear case, weak premises, the wrong premises? Remember that your coursework will often need to include arguments, so what you test out here could be especially valuable.

As this answer is based on your own observation, there is no outline answer at the end of the chapter.

Interpreting and speculating

Interpreting involves making sense of that which is encountered. A variety of stimuli are received by the nurse (e.g. auditory and visual information) and these are converted into perceptions (impressions) when the nurse combines this information with past experiences (memories). Successful interpretation then relies upon being alert to all of the possible information, and then understanding how this can be combined to determine what is happening (Cooper and Frain, 2016). Sometimes conflicting information will be encountered that makes it harder for the nurse to decide what the information signals (e.g. risk, improvement, deterioration, sepsis, a new stage of illness). Nevertheless, interpreting is an important skill element because it links enquiry to the formulation of the templates that you have already read about. Eventually, enough information might amass, tested against research and experience, for the nurse to say that there is a clear pattern which represents 'patient anxiety'. This is important, and we must act in these ways if patients are not to suffer unduly.

While searching for such patterns is most readily related to clinical demands, it is also important in your campus studies. A literature search may, for instance, suggest that recurring themes arise on your chosen topic. Imagine that you were investigating disfigurement and its effect on patient well-being. If the literature repeatedly threw up the importance of injury context (e.g. an acid attack) for the degree of distress that a disfigurement causes, it would be reasonable to highlight that in your analysis. We search for patterns of information to help determine where we enquire next and how we might respond.

I have left **speculation** until last, and I consider it extremely important. Successful nursing relies in large part on nurses 'thinking outside the box', daring to consider options or solutions that are unfamiliar. Creativity and imagination therefore form a valuable part of critical thinking, one that can help nurses to improve the lot of patients.

Sue talks about a nurse that she admired:

> *One specialist nurse I knew pulled all the information together about teaching diabetic patients, and she quickly realised that with the staff available they couldn't do it in the usual one-to-one way. That was when she suggested that they should teach patients in groups and organise the sessions so that the patients could help each other out. As the patients assisted one another, the specialist nurse watched them to assess who understood diet and insulin therapy.*

Remaining ready to speculate suggests an inquisitive mind and is welcomed by tutors. Here are some questions to consider that help you practise speculation:

> What is happening here?
>
> What is important if this happens?
>
> Why did that happen or unfold in that particular way?
>
> Why does this person seem upset or especially pleased?
>
> How did that process work (who did what, when and why?)
>
> Now that this has happened what could helpfully happen next?
>
> When will things change? (for example, the patient entering a new stage of illness?)
>
> Simple questions such as when, where, how, what and why help you develop an inquisitive and a speculative mind.

A readiness to speculate about what is problematic, or what could be done better or differently to make the best use of the resources available, is often at the heart of high-quality healthcare. Even when others prefer to work within the status quo, it is incumbent upon nurses to examine what is being done – and what more could be done – to improve patient care (Bolton and Delderfield, 2018).

How can we reason better?

Let us take stock. So far, we have acknowledged that critical thinking is important because of the challenging healthcare environment which you will work within. We have defined critical thinking as an inquisitive but disciplined process that involves human experiences and feelings, as well as empirical information. We have suggested what the key components are within critical thinking (e.g. deciding what can be claimed) and acknowledged the aptitudes that you will need to develop (e.g. asking questions) in order to succeed. I have suggested that learning involves incremental work towards templates, that which enables us to work effectively and efficiently to address nursing care needs. What seems effortless to the experienced nurse seems difficult for us because we are still developing our thinking skills.

At this stage, it is tempting to hope for a formula, a sure-fire way to think in the right way. Would that we could use that formula to write our essays. Unfortunately, there is no neat formula that encapsulates critical thinking in every circumstance. You will need to reason in different ways at different times, and sometimes combine information from your different places. In the past, nurses used to be taught bundled information (e.g. surgical nursing, medical nursing), but that did not facilitate the sort of nimble reasoning which nurses need today. We should not trap information in different silos relating to, for instance, cancer. That which we learn about coping, for example, may serve in many other contexts.

Nimble reasoning seems to work in two ways, sometimes in parallel:

- *Deductively*: We test theory (our own and that received) to see whether what we predict is in fact the case (e.g. concerning how people usually cope with illness).
- *Inductively*: We gather information in order to formulate theories of what is happening (e.g. noticing that patients tell stories about their illness as a means of managing stress levels).

Not all critical thinking is equal. There are certainly weaker and stronger ways of reasoning, and this usually informs how tutors mark coursework. The more sophisticated your reasoning approach, the better the mark you might attain. Rest assured, though, that expectations regarding your reasoning ability grow incrementally over the course – you are not expected to be an expert at the outset.

Reasoning approach	Description
Independent reasoning	We construct a template that adequately explains what is important about the work that we do. Perhaps that explains successful care: the nurse marries what the patient believes they need with what science recommends. We take a *position* on what is then important.
Contextual reasoning	We rely strongly on contexts to determine what we focus upon and accept that as important and valuable. For example, we might suggest that the social circumstances of the family of a dying patient strongly influence how they cope with the news that the illness is incurable.
Transitional reasoning	Reasoning involves living with doubts, about what is true, or important. We learn to wait and see, and accept that right now several explanations of the situation might have to be considered. We admit what we don't yet know.
Silent absorption	We absorb and appreciate a growing volume of information, noting the same without necessarily venturing an opinion. For example, perhaps you attend a series of lectures on infection, venturing no opinion on what is discussed until the series is complete.
Absolute reasoning	We search for what is right or wrong, making clear distinctions – that which is fact and that which is not. We search for the definitive answer that properly supports care decisions.

Table 1.2 Ways of reasoning

Activity 1.7   Decision-making

Look now at the array of reasoning described in Table 1.2. Decide which you think are the more sophisticated forms and which are much more basic. Decide for yourself if you employ one of these approaches more than others.

1. Absolute reasoning

Nursing demands different forms of reasoning at different times, but here I venture the following. The least sophisticated forms of reasoning are what Baxter Magolda (1992) calls *absolute* (Mason, 2005). At this level, the individual is unable to see the different nuances of a situation or accept that a range of possible perspectives could be taken on a subject. The thinker looks for certainty and only feels secure when matters have been decisively concluded (e.g. 'this is right', 'that is wrong', 'this is what we believe', 'that is what we don't believe'). If you are prone to thinking in this way, you might note how often you ask your tutor or practice supervisor to confirm what is 'correct'. While an absolute might be expected with regard to some areas of work (e.g. the right drug to use in an emergency), it is not something that is possible or even desirable in many other situations (e.g. finding the right way to deal with a hallucinating patient). **Absolute thinking** is a common way of reasoning at the start of a university education, and it is the least sophisticated because we expect rules to govern so many things.

2. Silent absorption

I have placed silent absorption next, as it is linked so strongly to inactivity. The thinker waits, soaking up more and more information in the hope that reasoning will be assisted by the accumulation of knowledge. In practice, this does not always work out, even though it may have been your tried-and-tested way of learning before. More information does not always lead to clarity, and there is a need to ask questions and discuss ideas if we are to develop confidence in our reasoning. Staying at the back of a class and hoping to avoid debates and discussions is not the best way to learn to reason, although it is understandable to begin with if the subject is entirely new to you.

3. Transitional reasoning

I suggest that transitional reasoning is better. The thinker is ready to live with the uncertainties of knowledge but is also ready to question as opportunities present themselves. You will need to reason in this way, accepting that in some clinical contexts, and for the time being, not all can be understood about a situation. Insights emerge from what is experienced and discussed, and in the meantime, it is necessary to remain alert to what experience or a carefully selected question can assist you with. You might be using transitional reasoning if you habitually try out questions with your tutor to clarify what seems acceptable in an essay.

4. Contextual reasoning

Contextual reasoning is even more sophisticated and suggests that the thinker understands there are lots of different truths in the world – and what works in one context does not always work in another. This is not to suggest that you have no principles or standards, or that 'anything goes' within nursing. Principles and safe practice are important, but there may well be different ways of doing things within those parameters. A good example of this working well is where nurses explore with patients the nature of dignity. What represents dignified care can vary widely, and take into account patient expectation, lifestyle and customs (Blomberg et al., 2019).

5. Independent reasoning

Independent reasoning is arguably the most sophisticated form of reasoning and one that helps you to become more innovative over time. At this level, you allow others to adopt their own position and to develop arguments in support of the same, while you build your own case about the subject in hand. You carefully search what there is to support your own position, stand ready to change it if others can persuade you, and treat all discussion in a thoughtful and enquiring way.

As you review your answer to Activity 1.7, do not be alarmed if your own thinking was near the bottom of this hierarchy. Students frequently need to work from the bottom. Moving from more familiar ways of reasoning to those that involve greater uncertainty and challenge means that you have to move out of your comfort zone.

Stewart, one of the case study students, described how his reasoning was slowly moving up the hierarchy described here. For him what was key was his own curiosity about a subject matter (e.g. patient psychology) and a 'found soul' that was adept at speculating about the subject with him. Two people in particular helped Stewart: a staff nurse on the ward and his personal tutor. Both helpers saw learning as fun and mistakes in thinking quite normal. What seems important is working with others whom you trust to respect your learning journey. Tutors are trained in such work but there are many others with an empathetic instinct for helping too. Such individuals typically:

- Demonstrate introspection, they question themselves and their ideas as they proceed.
- Have a sense of humour, smiling at their own small mistakes while focusing firmly on what must change.

- Play 'what if' games, imagining how situations could change, if the nurse proceeded differently.
- Use questions gently; they encourage you to revisit a claim, to explore an assumption.

You might think that only people at the pinnacle of the hierarchy of reasoning can help you make progress. This isn't entirely true though. Sometimes a subject expert is not necessarily so well versed in explaining their thinking to others. You might encounter awesome lecturers ('they know so much!'), who are inaccessible thinkers. The lecturer explains 'what' without necessarily explaining 'why'. So clever might they seem that you fear seeming stupid if you ask a question. What is important is that the person who helps you, understands the journey you are making. Great tutors and course designers do. Because learning is a discovery process too, where mistakes are allowed, it is perfectly possible to learn with and from another considerate student.

Learning in groups, with and from peers, is a valuable learning process. It's unwise to assume that only the qualified can teach you something. In turn you as well might find yourself helping a colleague learn. We hope that learning might be fun, but in truth, it is often a process of challenges and sudden relief as we take each step forward. When you experience that relief with a colleague, discover what you have both understood, it can seem the best experience.

Chapter summary

I have introduced you to basic ideas about critical thinking and explained that it is a process which involves the gathering, receiving and processing of information in order to understand the world around you. It is important in nursing for a number of reasons, e.g. problem-solving, and the management of a great deal of uncertainty that attends patient care.

Critical thinking has different components that you will meet again and again. You will, for instance, debate what can reasonably be asserted on a given topic. To do that, you will need to develop a series of aptitudes that will help you to advance your enquiries and make more confident decisions, such as asking the right questions.

While this can seem confusing, the purpose of your enquiries has in fact a logical and a professional end. You are learning to develop templates, ways of reasoning that work in practical and professional ways to deliver care to patients. While experienced nurses seem to do this effortlessly, they have in fact struggled much like you in the past. They have learned to identify patterns of information that serve them well when they deal with the ambiguity of care. There is a purpose to your learning: to respond to care requirements in an efficient, effective and patient-supportive way.

Learning to think critically, though, does not happen overnight. The nursing course is designed to exercise you in different activities that help you to move from more rigid ways of thinking towards nimble and innovative ones. Learning to think critically involves some anxiety, but expert tutors and practice supervisors are well versed in helping you to find a way through.

Activities: brief outline answers

Activity 1.1   Reflection (page 10)

Because the world of nursing is complex, information rich and sometimes contradictory it means that the subject cannot simply be instructed. Much as we might cherish a traditional lecture by an expert, that is unlikely by itself to equip us to think and act in ways that nursing requires. We will have to deal with the untidiness of nursing and the stressful demands made there. So, learning at university is likely to require much more active enquiry and collaboration. You are going to have to manage uncertainty more than in say in an academic subject previously taught at school. What can or should we do, where, how and why?

Activity 1.3   Reflection (page 14)

Here is my example. I think that we must be able to assert what counts as teaching. That might surprise you because you are learning to nurse, not to become a teacher. Yet I suggest that you will teach a great deal, especially to patients and relatives. Of course, teaching is different in clinical practice; we do not lecture patients and they are not put through exams like campus students. But we do have to help them solve problems, cope better and master medications. Knowing how teaching works, what we need to do to help patients adapt seems to me very important. It may determine whether patients stay safe and become independent again. A good understanding of teaching is of immediate benefit to practice – it has utility.

Activity 1.4   Reflection (page 14)

My memorable decision relates to helping patients recover from burns. I specialised in body image care. This patient, like many others, had facial burns and was anxious about encountering others who might stare at him. He was a Falklands War veteran who later became a public speaker, but he did not have much confidence back then. The patient and I debated how to get used to public settings again. We reviewed the merits of doing this on a 'try it and see' short-exposures basis. I suggested that he go to watch the news, sitting at the back of the ward TV room first. That was a legitimate reason to be out and about from his room but a short enough time not to become too uncomfortable. Other patients would also be focused primarily on the TV screen. I suggested that we treat it like a military exercise, with a debrief to discuss how it went at the end. We realised that to begin too quickly with more adventurous visits, perhaps to a shop or a café beyond the hospital, would seem too much. The decision, then, was a carefully consulted one, something that offered the patient options about what we might do next. I suspect that many of yours will be too. Nurses help patients to make decisions of their own.

Further reading

Braithwaite J (2006) *Critical thinking, logic and reason: a practical guide for students and academics.*

Don't be put off by the age of this article, it still offers valuable information about how reasoning is sometimes conceived of at university. You are likely to encounter scientists there who see reasoning strongly in Socratic terms. In nursing, however, we give greater scope to emotional intelligence. Braithwaite offers a good summary of reasoning and logic, a natural sciences complementary account to how I have conceived of critical thinking here.

Chatfield, T (2022) *Critical thinking: your essential guide*, 2nd edition. London: Sage.

This is a valuable book once you start to develop your own reasoning ability. It would work especially well when studying a postgraduate course. It is informative, too, if you are interested in the philosophical basis of reasoning, that taught by Socrates and others. Tom explores different contexts of reasoning, for instance scrutinising the arguments of others and detecting bias. He is writing for a wide student audience so don't expect healthcare application, but the more you become intrigued by reasoning, the more valuable this resource starts to seem.

Standing, M (2023) *Clinical judgement and decision making in nursing*, 5th edition. London: Sage/Learning Matters.

Mooi Standing details what underpins so much of clinical decision-making: the ways in which critical judgements are made in practice. This book provides an important illustration of applied critical thinking, drawing on ethics and evidence, as well as experience.

Useful websites

Note: Website material is subject to change or removal at short notice.

https://www.academia.edu/316239/Critical_Thinking_Logic_and_Reason_A_Practical_Guide_for_Students_and_Aca

Braithwaite J (2006) Critical thinking, logic and reason: a practical guide for students and academics.

Don't be put off by the age of this article, it still offers valuable information about how reasoning is sometimes conceived of at university. You are likely to encounter scientists there who see reasoning strongly in Socratic terms. In nursing, however, we give greater scope to emotional intelligence. Braithwaite offers a good summary of reasoning and logic, a natural sciences complementary account to how I have conceived of critical thinking here.

www.wikiHow.com/Reason

How to reason: 9 steps (with pictures)

This is certainly not an extensive review of reasoning in the full, but I do think that it offers a reassurance when your course of studies seems daunting. It breaks reasoning down into nine steps, I would call them working principles, that should help sustain your efforts. Among these is the need to suspect that which you feel quickly passionate about. We can quickly forget how deep-seated beliefs can sway us, without adequate thought. Also valuable were the remarks about imagining how others think or feel, that will stand you in good stead within nursing.

Chapter 2   Reflecting

(Continued)

Platform 5: Leading and managing nursing care and working in teams

At the point of registration, the registered nurse will be able to:

5.10 Contribute to supervision and team reflection activities to promote improvements in practice and services.

Chapter aims

After reading this chapter, you will be able to:

- define reflection, indicating how a stated purpose can help to make reflections more critical;
- distinguish the differences between reflecting in practice and reflecting on practice, detailing why they are different from one another;
- identify six reasons why reflection is important in nursing;
- discuss the best principles of reflection, identifying how you will proceed in the future.

Introduction

Nursing is strongly associated with the skill of reflection, and for good reason. Without adequate reflection, insight and **empathy**, it would be hard to see how the needs of the individual could be adequately addressed (Price, 2022). Without reflection, it would be difficult to see how imaginative, supportive and responsive care could be delivered over the course of a nursing career. Nurses need to understand themselves while learning to nurse, and they need to respect themselves while continuing to deliver safe care under exacting circumstances (Van Humbeeck et al., 2020).

Purposeful reflection

While reflection is a key skill within nursing, it is not necessarily easily mastered. This is in large part because we are all accustomed to reflecting in an ad hoc way. Nursing practice reflection needs to be better organised than that. Idle curiosity is not enough. Professional reflection needs to be characterised by several features.

First, professional reflection should have a clear purpose, one that relates to the context of your practice (Grant et al., 2017). However appealing it is to reflect in a free-ranging way, this risks confusion if the purpose of your reflection is not clear from the start. The following are some purposes that you might have for reflecting:

- To ascertain whether something represents a problem, and if so to determine why it has come about.
- To understand the process of something, such as how clinicians and families negotiate care.
- To help build working templates for future practice. It is a good idea, for example, to cluster reflections around themes, such as pain management. Reflections may then not only be individually more effective, but they may broaden your insight into care.
- To ascertain our strengths and weaknesses, that which sustains and motivates us in practice. Historically, reflections have been wedded to the adequacy of care, whether what you did was right. I would suggest that this is too narrow a focus. It can leave you feeling embattled and less enthusiastic about reflecting in the future.

Fatima, one of the case study students, shared with me her early doubts about reflecting on strengths and weaknesses. At the start of her course, she felt loaded with weaknesses. So, we sat down with Sue, the registered nurse, and she recounted her doubts several years after graduating. Doubt is normal; we will always doubt something about best practice and what we do. Indeed, without such doubt we might never improve. Over the course of Fatima's studies, the balance of strengths and weaknesses changed, and she grew in confidence. It was quite acceptable to doubt.

Second, professional reflection should be disciplined (Esterhuizen, 2022). A number of reflective practice models have been developed, setting out steps to follow. Some of those are complex, with a dozen or more questions to work through. My recommendation is to utilise the simplest model possible, one that asks questions such as what, so what and what next (MTa Learning, 2021; Rolfe et al., 2011). A good model allows you to set out the context of the episode, what happened and what you concluded (see Table 2.1). If you wish to reflect to a good standard it is necessary to ask one or more colleagues to reflect with you, challenging some of the ideas that you develop. It is only by speculating with others that you will be able to fine-tune the components of critical thinking which you read about in Chapter 1.

Question	Notes
What?	Set a context for your reflection, what happened and what people said or did. Note any thematic focus that prompted your interest here. Don't analyse yet, simply describe events.
So what?	Next describe why this seemed important and what seemed to influence proceedings. What was at issue, problematic, rewarding or intriguing? It's useful to examine how you thought different individuals approached the event (see Figure 2.1).
What next?	Summarise what you changed or believe needs to change in the future. Once again there is scope here to reflect on any important narratives or discourses that you identified.

Table 2.1 A Three Question Framework for Reflection (adapted from Rolfe et al., 2011)

The third feature of professional reflection relates to determining an appropriate scale for your work. The students who have influenced this book all attested to times when they attempted individual reflections that were poorly focused. You will help to manage the scale of reflection by having a clear purpose for each of them. So, for example, you might identify a purpose of understanding patient rehabilitation and then pick up on reflective practice episodes that fit there. Perhaps the first concerned a patient who resented the guidance of nurses. The second reflection centred on judging how much to coach a patient. A third reflection might centre on what happened when rehabilitation goals changed. Each of the individual reflections are discrete, but incrementally they can build something both larger and more informative. If you simply reflect indiscriminately, then you risk creating an explosion of possible ideas, those that increase doubt before you are ready to identify better solutions.

Reflection and time

Now, what about reflection and time. How does passing time affect the nature of reflection?

Activity 2.1   Reflection

Consider this statement: 'It is easier to reflect after the event rather than during it.'

- Do you support this argument?
- What supports your position?

At the end of the chapter, I share an observation or two of my own.

Schön (1987) believes that reflecting *on* action is different from reflecting *in* action. If we reflect on the event as it unfolds, we have none of the benefits of calm introspection and time to consider at leisure the different options available to us. Conversely, if we reflect long after the event, it is likely that our memory may play tricks on us, and we may remember certain features of the event better than others. Reflecting in practice involves 'thinking on our feet' (Edwards, 2017). We cannot pause the action, producing the sage-like response that we would love to deliver. Reflecting in action is 'raw', but it is perhaps vivid because of that. We can illustrate this with two short excerpts of reflection from Sue. In the first extract, Sue is reflecting in action, and in the second she is reflecting on action. It is important to note that in-action reflections are usually unspoken – speaking aloud our thoughts could prove problematic in many clinical settings.

In the following episode Sue has encountered a potentially aggressive relative.

Case study: Reflection in action and reflecting on action

Reflecting in action

Is this man going to hit me? He seems angry. What does he want? I need to say something, do something that shows him I respect his concerns. I need to suggest something. I know, I'll suggest that we talk in the relatives' room but leave the door open in case I need assistance. That shows I will give him time to tell me what worries him, and I'll remain safe. Yes, that seems to have worked, he is agreeing to accompany me. But he's still talking as we go. He's like a pressure cooker, and I'm worried about how that will seem to the other relatives on the ward.

Reflecting on action

The relative had suffered a major shock. He thought he had nearly a week to prepare for his wife to come home, but she was to be discharged that afternoon. No wonder he was upset. We were meeting our needs to make a bed available for someone else but returning the patient back into his care at short notice. Colleagues could see that his wife required some more rehabilitation at home, so care would be complex.

The above excerpts show just how different reflecting seems at these points. Notice the staccato way in which thoughts emerge when reflecting in action. There is an urgent search for meaning. Sue must work with her perceptions of what the relative is feeling, as well as her own experiences of a confrontation. The reflections on action, however, are evaluative and confident, as well as indicating considerable empathy for the man. Sue can assert a great deal more about the origins of the problem. The important point here is that reflecting in action is necessarily less considered, less perfect than that which is possible afterwards.

In your nursing course or later as part of revalidation, you will be asked to prepare reflective practice written work. Demonstrating your powers of reflection is important. There are different levels of reflection, however – something that we discuss further in Chapter 3. What is usually sought is critical reflection, which is harder to achieve if you reflect in practice (Esterhuizen, 2022). Role-played care can simulate – to differing degrees – reflection in action, but most assessment invites you to reflect on practice retrospectively. Critical reflection requires you to take an overview and understand how your own values, beliefs and goals affect the way in which you approach patients, and how that in turn interacts with how they feel and what they might wish to achieve. It is much harder to 'see the bigger picture' in the middle of healthcare events.

In your course, the opportunities to reflect on practice may be legion. You will be asked to write reflective essays and develop case studies that explore the quality of care delivered to patients. Price (2017) explains how reflective practice case studies can link experience and evidence together. Opportunities to reflect in action and with support are much rarer. If you are fortunate, they will occur with an experienced practice supervisor who can help you to rehearse aloud your thinking within a psychologically safe environment, that is, where a reflective account does not alarm patients (O'Sullivan et al., 2021).

It is important here to think about the sequence of events. You are likely to encounter a mass of clinical and other events (those on campus count too), which might be worthy of reflection. Manifestly, though, it is unrealistic to reflect on everything – you would quickly become exhausted. So, begin by contemplating what seems significant about your experiences. Do they relate closely to the objectives of your current module of study? Do they relate to one of your reflective purposes, perhaps something about a skill that you feel less certain about? By selecting reflections to concentrate upon, you are likely to write fewer but much better developed reflections. It is often the quality of reflection rather than the quantity of reflective records that will help to secure your progress.

Working with accounts, narratives and discourses

Nurses encounter others' behaviour, perhaps a hug, shake of the fist, or smile, and then we try to interpret that. But we also listen to an *account* of others' experiences, feelings or attitudes (e.g. 'I'm livid that my wife has to come home from hospital so soon!'). Lying beneath that account, and either more or less coherently expressed, there may be a *narrative* – an underlying story that the individual uses to make sense of what is happening and what they are trying to accomplish (Aasen et al., 2021). In this instance, the relative's narrative might relate to requesting more discharge preparation time. The whole encounter, though, may be part of a bigger storyline – a *discourse* – which is something that helps to explain what is under way, that deemed normal or desirable (Fjortoft et al., 2020). The obvious discourse here concerns discharge planning and lay care liaison. Discourses must usually take account of your goals, values and attitudes. When encountering an aggressive patient for example, you will do so with some attitudes already present. It is unreasonable to assault a nurse; we are caring staff. But angry people do not behave rationally, so it's important to stay safe. What we really want to achieve here is a win–win situation – one where the relative feels respected, and we can find a solution to the problem of discharging the patient from hospital. Stakeholders within a discourse might disagree vehemently about what is under way and what should happen. Figure 2.1 illustrates how these elements might fit together.

What marks out our care from other healthcare professionals such as doctors is that we work so intimately with the feelings, perceptions and hopes of those we support. We work with the patients' minds and emotions. This is emotionally taxing but is what distinguishes a very skilful nurse from someone who operates more as a technician.

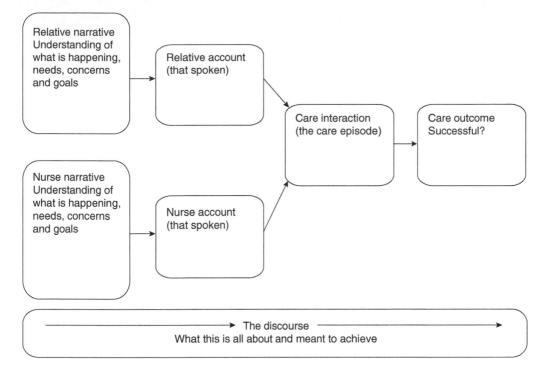

Figure 2.1 Accounts, narratives and discourses

It is because of this focus of our work that we reflect upon the accounts shared (ours and theirs), the narratives (explanations) used by interested parties, and the discourses in play (what people think should happen, that which is judged normal or desirable).

What you learn about narratives and discourses in care is going to become very important to you. But it takes time to identify these in others or indeed to examine our own narratives and discourses. It is difficult to be sure what you have witnessed. You are naturally cautious. But with time, observations in clinical practice and discussion through seminars, you will develop growing confidence in interpreting what you see and hear. How do patients usually respond to the challenge of rehabilitation for example? What do they find difficult? What within what we say or how we act seems to support and encourage them?

Activity 2.2   Reflection

To help you to explore these new terms jot down now what you think should characterise the rehabilitation of a patient (what is normal or desirable). This is your starting discourse (the patient and relatives may have their own). Next, jot down what sorts of narratives might exercise the patient or relative, that which tests your discourse. How might you identify those narratives in play (the accounts)?

My brief answer to this is given at the end of this chapter.

Defining reflection

Now that you have begun to explore what reflection involves, we can venture a definition:

> *Reflection is a process whereby experience is examined in ways that give meaning to interaction. We might examine the experience in real time or in retrospect. Because experience engages the emotions as well as reasoning, reflection needs to take account of the feelings engendered within an interaction and to allow that perceptions may sometimes prove erroneous. Reflection may be used in the service of different purposes – those that help us to think in a more critical way and to serve the ethos of nursing. Through an analysis of accounts, narratives and discourses, reflection helps the nurse to better understand the nature of others' needs and concerns. It may also acquaint the nurse with that which they find taxing in practice, something that must be understood if nursing is to be a lifelong career.*

Why reflection is important

Figure 2.2 represents some of the reasons why reflection is so important in nursing. Your appreciation of the value of reflection is likely to grow the further you progress through your course.

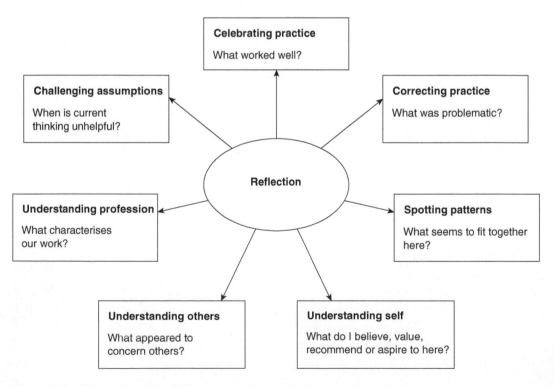

Figure 2.2　Why reflection is important in nursing

Spotting patterns

Reflection is important because it helps us to spot patterns of behaviour, combinations of evidence, and cause-and-effect events that are important in nursing (Barratt, 2019). The patterns that you might spot arise not only in clinical practice, but in classrooms and lectures as well. Themes seem to emerge and reoccur. Let me share one example with you. My clinical practice first centred on trauma. I looked after patients with burns, gunshot wounds, and bomb blast and road traffic accident injuries. Later I worked in cancer care.

What was common to all the above care areas was psychological trauma. Patients had to come to terms with changes to their appearance, as well as their body's functions and reliability. That in which they lived (the body) might not remain as comfortable or dependable as they first thought. I started to note that patients recovering from different injuries, operations and treatments seem to centre their emotional work in three areas (Price, 2016):

- managing how their body is now (the physical challenge);
- revising ideals about their body and appearance or function (the body and self-esteem);
- finding ways to address the discrepancies between their body ideal and how it in fact looks or works.

I named the three areas of work. The first, I called 'body reality' (the body as diseased, injured or changed). The second I called 'body ideal' (how the individual hoped that the body would seem or function). The third I called 'body presentation' (how the body is arranged, dressed and presented, that which supports self-esteem). I was then able to use those ideas to review and improve my care work. So, for example, I might help a patient to rehearse new ways of thinking about themselves after a burn. What were their other attributes beyond appearance? Did people value their sense of humour, their intelligence for example? Care was then centred on helping them to appreciate and represent themselves in a wider range of ways.

Do you see how spotting patterns within practice, what challenges patients, became a process of grouping information and turning that into a new way of caring? Spotting patterns of information, behaviour, need and reaction to others assists you to theorise and formulate better templates of care. While this altered body image reasoning developed over years and was large-scale, it does still illustrate the process under way. If you do not spot patterns in this way, care can become formulaic.

Activity 2.4   Planning

Jot down now one or two themes of interest that you would like to reflect upon when you next encounter patients in clinical practice. Why are you interested in those? Speculatively, what do you imagine might be discovered there? Good themes to choose are those that many patients might exhibit which have practical importance for how you deliver care. These might include understanding their illness, managing treatment, asking for help or explaining their worries. The recommended reflective practice model on your course will suggest a series of questions to guide your reflection, but do not be afraid to ponder any recurring points that seem to arise from several different patients. Was a pattern forming?

As this answer is based on your own observation, there is no outline answer at the end of the chapter.

Celebrating practice

Reflection on action can be put to excellent use to celebrate and explain practice that is successful (Calhoun and Esparza, 2017). It is not enough for nurses to simply pat themselves on the back for a job well done. We need to understand how we brought about the desirable outcomes. It is easy to underestimate the value of reflection used in this role, but within a stressful healthcare environment it is vital. It is vital that nurses celebrate success as well as review problems and shortfalls. As you reflect on what has worked especially well in care, it is also important to consider what counts as success. Do we mean more effective care (greater impact), more efficient care (better use of resources), more sensitive care (working with the needs of patients) or more collegiate care (working better with other professions)?

Gina in particular values this role of reflection. She reports that in the very best care teams the nurses confidently report what they have achieved and that they are then better at assessing plans within a multidisciplinary team. As she put it, 'nurses must know what they bring to the table'.

Correcting practice

Reflection is frequently used to determine what went wrong and what was problematic. *In extremis*, it may be used to determine who we believe was to blame for untoward events. Reflection is employed, for instance, as part of a root cause analysis (searching for the origins of a problem) in cases where there have been shortfalls in clinical decision making (Gurlay et al., 2021). Root cause analysis gives focus to reflection and sharpens critical awareness of what went wrong. Reflecting in this way, on what was problematic or erroneous, is difficult. It is emotionally taxing to confront what we believe were our mistakes, as well as what we might have done better or differently. If the nurse works in a culture where individuals are scapegoated (blamed exclusively for a problem shaped by many more professionals) then reflection might be hotly contested. Just what did go wrong and what contributed to that? What didn't we understand or appreciate?

In some instances, what counts as a problem might seem relatively self-evident. For example, if the patient received the wrong drug and was adversely affected, then that is problematic. But in some other areas of care, the decision on what represents a problem might be complex. Imagine an anxious set of parents who believe that a particular treatment might significantly improve the quality of life of their terminally sick child. For these parents, it is problematic if the clinical team do not provide that treatment. Expert evidence is called upon. The problem is then that the definitions of both 'problem' and 'solution' become disputed. Sometimes, then, reflection is used to understand why there are competing views and why the debate is stressful for all concerned.

Reflecting on what seems problematic is easier with a mentor. This individual explores with you your perceptions of events and helps you to examine the conclusions that you reach. How big a problem was this? Why did it occur? What were your options? What decisions were important here? What are the pluses as well as the minuses of the course of action that you chose? As part of her preparation work for revalidation of her practice, Sue (our case study registered nurse) described the help that she got:

> *My practice supervisor was perfect as she uses the word 'because'. She might say, 'I think that situation was a problem because the team were making different assumptions about care.' She might say, 'I think you're wrong to chastise yourself over that because the patient was very ambiguous about what they already understood about their illness.' You only benefit from reflection when it gets linked to reasoning, and a word as simple as 'because' facilitates that.*

Remember (from Chapter 1), what distinguishes an argument from mere opinion is the addition of underlying premises, that which underpins what you say (Price, 2019a). This is why the word 'because' is especially important when building an argument, presenting a discourse on how you see nursing care before you.

Understanding self

In some areas of nursing (e.g. mental health, palliative care), an understanding of our motives and values is especially important because we use ourselves to therapeutic purpose. Our ability to share personal insights, or to imagine how others feel, may be critical (Outlaw et al., 2018). The ability to empathise, for example, becomes integral to entering the world of the patient and their anxieties, but one that must be managed with a certain detachment if professional judgements are to remain sound. A successful nurse builds an excellent rapport with patients and empathises with their concerns, but also manages to adopt a position where they can later challenge some of the patients' unhelpful beliefs.

These are important points and may be the focus for some of your study interests. If you think of nursing in craft terms, your emphasis is likely to be on skills and the way that these are selected and applied. However, if you think of nursing in more aesthetic terms, you are likely to feel more comfortable reflecting on your values and beliefs, precisely because you see these as essential to delivering the best care. In recent years, and under considerable healthcare service pressures, the values of nurses have come under increasing scrutiny. It is no longer taken for granted that nurses have a vocation and will instinctively do the right thing.

I asked Fatima about this role of reflection, and she made a very important point. It's likely that as you move between different clinical placements that notions of what is most important in nursing changes. Nurses value themselves in different ways. In areas such as intensive or high dependency care for example the focus is typically on skills. In mental health care areas though the nurse seems to focus on something else. She called it 'supportive companionship'. It was compassionate to listen, to be a supportive presence for distressed patients. Sometimes there wasn't a particular thing to do, a solution to be applied. The nurse could not complete the work that the patient themselves needed to do.

Understanding others

Much of nursing is concerned with assisting others. Person-centred care assumes that we can successfully ascertain the patient's worries, needs and aspirations as a key determinant of the negotiated nursing care (Price, 2022). If we are to practise sensitively, then we must understand people and their backgrounds. There are some problems, though, with using reflection to understand others – chief among these is what we might call the 'common sense' fallacy. We might take it as a given that people in a particular situation (e.g. when suffering pain) will wish to proceed as we would (i.e. to have that pain alleviated). We are at risk of imagining that our preferences and wishes are shared by others and neglecting a check on their views. Not all patients aspire to alleviate all of their pain; indeed, some may refuse pain relief measures altogether. A devout Buddhist, for example, might observe that pain has something to teach us, and to remove it entirely is unhelpful.

Reflection used to understand others is necessarily speculative and needs to accommodate what arises out of each situation. What is important here is the discovery of the other person's narrative, how they explain events to themselves. The fact that a person relies upon odd information, should not prompt the nurse to simply correct them. We must understand the process of the patient's reasoning. That narrative might be reinforced by family opinion or the assessment of lay carers, and it may seem entirely unscientific. Yet until the nurse understands how the other person reasons, no individualised support can really be offered. That which might at best be considered helpful could quickly be received as a 'busybody prescription'. Reflection in these circumstances might become collaborative, the nurse assisting the patient to review what they think is happening and what needs to be done next. Where factual errors are then identified, a careful correction can be made, but in most other instances the supportive and reflective stance is one of helping the other person determine what they think now.

Understanding the profession or service

It may surprise you to discover that reflection has a part to play in understanding your chosen profession and service. Part of what sustains you as a practitioner concerns clear ideas about what nurses do, what expertise they bring, and what is different about the practice of the nurse. These are important considerations in a healthcare world where nurses are asked to diversify the sorts of work they engage in and where financial or other constraints might shape what the nurse can achieve (Michalowsky et al., 2020). Raymet observed that sometimes nurse managers thought like a clinical nurse and sometimes like a quartermaster. Patients competed for scarce resources and the individual nurse had to be circumspect about what was promised. Nursing remains both a professional and an ethical activity: we cannot simply work without the goals and the resources of the service.

Challenging assumptions

Reflection plays a major role in changing practice and changing profession over time. Healthcare work is not static, but it evolves, and what was once seemingly ideal later becomes suspect and anachronistic. For example, if you were to read nursing textbooks from the 1960s, you would discover that nursing care was perceived simply as supplemental to medicine. Today, nurses are much more strategic and engage in the design of healthcare (Wilson et al., 2019).

One of the best uses of reflection, then, is at a conference or when reading a report or policy associated with nursing to ascertain: (a) whether this reflects your current understanding of best practice; and (b) whether, in the light of what you have encountered there, you need to change. Reflection in this context is often best conducted as part of a group of nurses, especially where local protocols or best practice guidelines are formulated. Working in concert with others, you are more likely to formulate an informed opinion and counterbalance the first negative emotional response that can arise when you are invited to change. As a student, you may have opportunities to join team meetings and discussion groups where just such reflections are under way.

Activity 2.5   Reflection

Pause now to review the different purposes of reflection. Did any surprise you or perhaps cause you some concern? People don't all find reflection equally comfortable as a process. Some are more private than others. Elements of reflection though will arise in most areas of your learning. Rest assured, reflection is not a ritualistic formula where you must think in a rigid way. Provided that you remain open to alternative ideas and further possibilities, reflection need not prove a threat to your progress. While you will face challenges (for example as regards what you believe) there remain avenues to build richer beliefs and values too.

As this is a personal reflection activity, no additional answer appears at the chapter end.

Making reflection work for you

It's time now to bring all the elements of reflection together and to recommend how you might use it during your studies. Table 2.2 sets out what I suggest, but it is important as well to consult your personal tutor. Universities may deploy reflection in different ways within your course.

Recommendation	Notes
Start with a clear, reflective purpose, a question or theme that helps guide your enquiries.	In order not to end up with a mass of unrelated or difficult to write reflections, it is a good idea to start with a theme. There is no 'right' number of reflections to complete, only clear evidence that you are discovering things from what you see and hear.
Reflect when you are fresh.	Reflection is often hard work and may provoke uncomfortable emotions. It is important to select the best times to reflect, when you feel emotionally calm, and where you have found the right space to conduct such work.
Identify confidantes with whom you are comfortable reflecting.	Choose reflective partners that you trust, not simply those who will affirm your opening assessments of events. If they say things such as 'Have you thought about …', then you have the right sort of partner.
Allocate sufficient time and attention for the enterprise.	Reflection is a meditative activity that requires as much thinking time as writing time. It is wise to allocate at least an hour to produce an inquisitive and coherent reflection.
Use a simple reflective model such as 'what, so what and what next?' (MTa, 2021). Add in insights regarding discourses, narratives and accounts.	Your course might prescribe a reflective framework to use but where you are free to choose, I commend simplicity and flexibility. These three questions allow you to explore discourses, narratives and accounts against questions two and three.

Recommendation	Notes
Create reflective records that you can use again.	To use reflective records later, you need to include enough contextual details to understand the events in question. Make sure that you remind yourself what was happening, when the events occurred, and what resources or support were available. Date the record to help you sense any changes in your perspective that occur over time.
In making and using such records, respect the rights of others.	In making reflective records, you necessarily refer to other people, so ensure that you make their names and roles anonymous. It is important to store records securely and ensure that you do not unfairly defame others. Read over your written reflections, as well as inviting others to do so, to reduce the risk that you are simply reinforcing past prejudices or assumptions.

Table 2.2   First principles of successful reflection

There are important points to make about Table 2.2. The first concerns wide-ranging reflection versus purposeful reflection. Some of the frameworks used by students to conduct and record their reflections focus solely on the episode itself. You might accumulate lots of unrelated reflective episode records. It is then more difficult to determine what you are discovering. Start with a purpose for your reflections. By exploring the accounts of patients, relatives and practitioners, those that could influence policy, you will be better placed to examine how nurses can improve care. This is especially important as part of revalidation work for qualified nurses. The NMC requires registered nurses to record evidence of their professional update activities (e.g. attendance at a conference), others' evaluations of care, and personal reflections on practice (NMC, 2019). A much more powerful case can be made about the nurse's fitness to practise when reflections connect two or more of the different elements together. So, for example, linking reflections to patient feedback on the quality of care is a good way of demonstrating the nurse's responsiveness to expressed patient need.

Activity 2.6   Group working

A useful reflective exercise is to focus on an area with which most of you have some experience. Most people have some experience of grief (e.g. a lost relative or friend, changed circumstances such as divorce, the loss of a pet), so this can be a good starting point from which to explore some themed reflections.

Start by individually cataloguing your perceptions of what grief is and what is needed in terms of support. Writing points down will help you to map the range of ways in which grief and support are understood.

(Continued)

(Continued)

Share your thoughts with the group. Do the points raised by others expand your understanding? If you noted some widely agreed points, does that give you confidence to start building some ideas as regards what constitutes human needs? If you collectively discover some patterns of information, so much the better.

As this answer is based on your own observation, there is no outline answer at the end of the chapter.

As well as thinking about how much time you allocate for reflecting, consider, too, the sequence of thinking and writing. In part, you are thinking even as you write, but this has the disadvantage that as your thoughts arrive on the page or screen, further thoughts – sometimes contradictory ones – are triggered: 'It could be this, it could be that.' 'This was important, but then again perhaps it was not.' Therefore, it seems beneficial to allow yourself thinking-only time, or perhaps 'think and jot ideas down' time, so you can play with the possibilities before you. While the final written reflection does not necessarily need to be highly polished, it should be sufficiently accessible and coherent for you to use it to revise your care later. For that reason, I advise thinking and drafting thoughts first, then penning refined reflective records later. Both spontaneous notes and final reflections can be recorded in your portfolio (offering a full audit trail of thought).

Activity 2.7   Research

Investigate which reflective framework is recommended in association with your course. Discuss with your tutor what is expected in association with each of the reflective model headings there, and whether the course permits any latitude regarding how you set out your records. Establish whether the recommended framework allows you to establish the purpose of your reflection, or whether you need to add this as a preliminary introduction.

As this answer is based on your own observation, there is no outline answer at the end of the chapter.

Table 2.2 sets out my recommended way of proceeding. If you follow these principles however you should notice that you are integrating the different elements of reflection into your studies. Reflection will seem purposeful and there is a greater chance that it meets one or more roles of reflection. Instead of amassing multiple ad hoc reflections you will have worked with themes that excite and motivate you. These are just the areas of study planning that I think will excite your personal tutor. Remember, completing a course of studies is not simply consuming all that is taught, it involves making some discoveries of your own. Proceeding in such a purposeful way and trusting selected others to discuss your ideas with you should incrementally help you to build confidence. Reflecting on that which motivates and intrigues you is much more likely to carry you through to final examinations. In my experience, working in this way, students do indeed start to build templates and good ideas for practice that they can share and test out with others.

Chapter summary

This chapter has explored reflection as a form of critical thinking, one that focuses upon experience and takes into account the emotions associated with experience, as well as an account of empirical events. Episodes of care are usefully connected to our understanding of narratives and discourses, that which shapes ideas about care and need. What do people value? What do they care most about? Particular emphasis is placed on organising reflections with a clear purpose and searching for emergent patterns that might guide your future studies and even prompt you to sketch out templates of what you think is needed in such care situations.

Reflection seems like two skills in one. If we reflect in action, we are thinking on our feet and reading practice situations as quickly and accurately as possible. If we reflect on action, we use the benefits of hindsight but need to beware that reflecting too long after an event can result in problems associated with memory. While it is unrealistic to analyse all experiences *in situ* (you would suffer from information overload), it is possible to accumulate reflections after events, increasing your insights into your motives and actions, as well as the consequences of what you do.

Activities: brief outline answers

Activity 2.1 Reflection (page 30)

It might not surprise you that I think reflecting after the event is easier than during it, provided that there is not too great a time lag until we reflect. To reflect on events from today or yesterday is viable, but to reflect on events from a month ago is more suspect because of memory. Here are the premises that inform my position:

1. During events, we often experience information overload, and that information comes in different forms: words, sights, sounds and touch. So, to process it, to assign it meaning, is so much harder.

2. When we are in the midst of practice, we are acting a role, playing a part. So, we have to attend to what we feel, say or do, as well as what others initiate, how they in turn react to us. Reading that amount of interaction is very difficult.

3. The way in which people communicate moment by moment is often ambiguous. We can only start to make sense of an episode when we begin to identify patterns of behaviour, sequences of things said. This is because we make sense of patient wholes rather than isolated fragments of behaviour. We are much more likely to identify those when reflecting back on events. Reflecting back, we may draw on other experiences to spot what seemed important.

Activity 2.2 Reflection (page 33)

My opening discourse on rehabilitation

Rehabilitation is a collaborative activity designed to increase the patient's confidence and self-care, and it is dependent upon motivating the patient to share in the measures agreed. Typically, rehabilitation involves some kind of learning, although the nurse might not be the sole teacher.

Rehabilitation requires sustained effort and setbacks might be met. For that reason, there may be the need to solve problems and revise goals en route. Rehabilitation works towards the patient's goals as well as what the nurse commends as important. Rehabilitation requires progress checks, 'how are we doing?'

Anticipated patient narratives

- To limit the perceived risks and costs of rehabilitation (that which seems daunting)
- To become incrementally more independent
- To sustain dignity while learning, demanding the respect of the nurse
- To secure as much help as possible, sustaining effort, especially at the start of rehabilitation.

Possible patient accounts

The patient may express fears, hopes and doubts en route and at times they might feel frustrated or angry. The patient might ask a great many questions and on occasion, insist that they would like to proceed in a different way (rehabilitation is negotiated). The patient might express relief and satisfaction as milestones are achieved, but at other times despair might be expressed.

Further reading

Boyd, C (2023) *Reflective practice for nurses.* Oxford: Wiley/Blackwell.

Claire Boyd sets out her teaching stall in three sections, introducing the reader first to what reflection is, next, the process of using reflection to learn and finally in section 3 a series of case studies illustrating reflection in practice. Post Covid-19, the clinical environment is an especially challenging environment within which to reflect and to deliver care. The case studies were particularly interesting then, exploring the ideal and the reality of practice.

Esterhuizen, P (2023) *Reflective practice in nursing,* 5th edition. London: Sage/Learning Matters.

This practical guide recommends the use of reflection in a range of settings, the development of more inquisitive and speculative approaches to nursing care, and ethical ways to make reflective practice records. The author has wide experience of delivering care both home and abroad. It's worth reflecting upon how culture helps shape the notion of care.

Useful websites

While there are a host of different reflective frameworks recommended by universities the three-question approach offers simplicity and a considerable degree of flexibility as you reflect on different topics and situations. Keeping it simple offers you scope to become more creative as well as critical in how you examine experience. Of course you will need to comply with any reflective frameworks set for assessment purposes, but see if the three-question approach gives you confidence to get going.

https://youtu.be/vGyjF9Ngd8Y

'What is critical reflection? Introducing the what, so what and now what model'. McLaughlin Library.

This YouTube video introduces you to the three-question approach and it is equally easy to understand. As before I'd recommend weaving in discussion of discourses, narratives and account to add a critical edge, but it's an excellent introduction.

Chapter 3 Scholarly writing

Chapter aims

After reading this chapter, you will be able to:

- summarise what we mean by scholarly writing, relating this to different levels of learning;
- discuss the key features of essay structure and how these facilitate your explanation of learning achieved to date;

(Continued)

(Continued)

- explore the ways in which past experiences of writing can shape assumptions about scholarly writing in the future;
- make a clear case for 'thinking time' when preparing to write an academic paper;
- identify areas within your own writing where there is future scope for development.

Introduction

Scholarly writing is not only a proof of learning (a product); it is also an exercise for the mind. We improve our reasoning, test our assumptions, and develop the templates we learned about in Chapter 1 through the process of writing and securing feedback. In the 1970s, Noel Burch emphasised the importance of this, describing the emotional work of learning (Adams, 2016; Young et al., 2019). He referred to a competence ladder. At the bottom of the ladder, writing alerts us to things that we do not understand and our skill deficits in dealing with that subject matter. The feedback we receive on writing highlights things that we have not attended to, that which has been misconstrued. Later, we build upwards from that keenly aware of our shortfalls in reasoning and written expression. With writing practice and good feedback, you become consciously skilled (i.e. learning how to reason and express ideas on paper in a consistently clear way). First, though, we must confront what we do not yet know. We traverse through a time when feedback tells us that much of our reasoning seems disorderly. Competence and then apparent innate writing ability, which article writers seem to manage so easily, is achieved only after the mechanics of reasoning and writing are well understood.

I start this chapter with three observations to reassure you. First, writing in a scholarly way is a relatively new skill for most students. Even though you may have written academic essays at school, it is less likely that these will also have been vocational, linking theory to practice. Within an undergraduate pre-registration nursing degree, your thinking and writing will need to progress through different levels. Personal tutors understand this, so you should make good use of them as the assessment requirements evolve over the course of your studies. It is not 'weak' to seek guidance on meeting the requirements of your assessments. Second, writing in a scholarly way can be successfully learned provided that you take a little time to consider the process of work before you. While there are several different writing formats used within nursing courses (e.g. writing reflectively, writing about theory), all are open to analysis, and students can and do improve their writing with practice. We will return to different formats of writing in Part 3.

Stewart, Fatima, Raymet and Gina (our case study nursing students) all concede that they find writing difficult. Stewart came to nursing from a career in commerce, where his writing was less reflective than is often required here. Fatima and Raymet note that they not only wrestle with writing in the required nursing form, but also with some of the conventions of academic discussion required in British universities. There were different traditions of writing where they studied before, in India and Botswana. Gina thinks that she begins with the clearest possible starting point as she is not used to any other tradition in writing. She has the most recent experience of secondary education. Their personal tutors have acknowledged the various challenges they all face, observing that students who move between one career, culture or educational system and another need help to adapt to the expectations of their new environment. Irrespective of which background students come from, then, new skills will have to be learned and past assumptions about writing reconsidered.

In this chapter, we will work with student experience and I will lead you through different aspects of scholarly writing. This involves the connection of critical thinking and reflection to the conventions of scholarly expression. We examine the ways in which you might best represent what you have reasoned and reflected upon. We begin this work with a brief but important introduction to different levels of learning that shape course design. Sometimes the expectations of learning in the first, second, third and fourth years of a course are difficult to distinguish from one another. Confusingly, coursework assessments may, for example, use some descriptors such as 'critically discuss' across levels of learning, so it is hard to determine what the examiners expect. However, to help you with discussions with your module leader and personal tutor, I venture my own framework describing levels of critical thinking and reflection that relate specifically to the applications of thinking discussed in Chapters 1 and 2. I use them here and in Part 3 to better illustrate how your thinking might become more sophisticated as a course progresses.

I next examine how best to prepare for writing. I discuss the basic structure of academic pieces of work. While this will vary depending upon the format of writing that you are asked to engage in, I believe that there are some opening tenets of good writing that can be learned here. Lastly, I discuss what we mean by academic voice (Price, 2003). Academic voice refers to what the student hopes to convey in a piece of writing. You are required to develop an independent and inquisitive voice, a style of writing that critically examines what others have claimed and venture afterwards considered arguments of your own. Understanding the style of writing required, the academic voice, will help you to write a more successful paper.

Levels of learning

While most students experience assessment work simply as a series of hurdles to be completed, universities structure work in a quite specific way. Less taxing assessments appear at the start of the course and more exacting ones towards the end. As the subject matter studied changes, this progression might not be quite so apparent to you. You may identify easy and hard subjects, which might effectively cloak what the educators are working to achieve. In principle, though, less exacting ways of thinking and reflecting are tolerated at the start of your studies, and then, when you have been taught more skills and have been practised in academic writing for longer, you are expected to demonstrate more sophisticated reasoning.

Activity 3.1 Reflection

Look back in your course handbook to see what learning outcomes have been set for your studies, and how these change as you progress from Year 1 to Year 2, and so on, through the programme of studies. Do the learning outcomes associated with the later modules of your study seem harder? Is there a greater emphasis on creativity and the ability to evaluate?

As this answer is based on your own observation, there is no outline answer at the end of the chapter.

I have been persuaded by Baxter Magolda's (1992) explanation of levels of reasoning, which offers a clear summary of how reasoning can progress. In the least sophisticated forms of reasoning, individuals are inflexible and rule governed, seeing only one explanation, one point of view. As reasoning becomes more sophisticated, it becomes first transitional (other possibilities are accommodated) and then contextual. The reasoning is nuanced, and it relates to a given set of circumstances. It is not that theories are not valuable; it is that they need to be understood in the context of need or use. Remember that in Chapter 1, I emphasised that it was important to discern how usable information is, whether it has practical utility (Dolan et al., 2022). To be a successful nurse, you need to appreciate that not all information applies everywhere. You need to develop a quizzical attitude towards that which is taught: Is this true? Does it apply in every context? Ideas may seem exciting, but in nursing ideas must work with the competing demands upon the nurse. That which seems possible might not be probable when we weigh up the goals that we try to achieve. McBee et al. (2018) explain just how powerful and important contextual influences are in the clinician's reasoning. Much of what we must understand and do is negotiated in context. There is often no absolute right answer in healthcare, only better ways forward. At the pinnacle of reasoning is independent thought. For our purposes, we can think of independent thinking as that which includes a vision for better practice, which shows the nurse 'thinking outside the box'. Independent thought reframes information in ways that enable the nurse to see problems or challenges afresh and to identify new opportunities.

We can link Baxter Magolda's (1992) levels of reasoning to the applications of critical thinking and reflecting, discussed in Chapters 1 and 2. I have combined these into two tables: one for critical thinking (Table 3.1) and one for reflection (Table 3.2). In studying these tables, you should anticipate that the highest-order critical thinking and reflections skills will develop in full during the later modules of your study. Contextual thinking, for example, cannot be anticipated until you have had the chance to try out ideas in practice. Independent thinking is often associated with project work, something that is classically used to complete a level of study or your degree as a whole. While this all might seem a little daunting, remember that we learn to reason better as part of a well-designed course. You are not expected to be an independent thinker from the outset.

	Absolute thinking (early learning)	Transitional thinking	Contextual thinking	Independent thinking (advanced learning)
Asking questions	Few or no questions asked, information accepted as fact.	Questions asked about whether claims are correct, whether other possibilities might exist.	Nuanced questions asked, those applying to a circumstance or need. Typically, these relate to a patient, plan or practice and its protocols.	Imaginative new questions are asked, those that reframe the topic, problem or issue in some way, liberating you to suggest fresh ideas.
Discriminating	There is little or no discrimination about what is right best or proven.	Knowledge is seen as contentious in some regard and open to debate. You write about why something may be preferred, with reference to values, evidence and goals.	Information is interrogated with regard to its fit within a circumstance or need. Theories are applied, and ideas are examined and combined with experience to explore what works.	Judgements on best information to use are now refined, articulating a range of influencing factors that you take into account.
Interpreting and speculating	At best, you select information to include in your report of what seems defensible, and practicable. Interpretation rarely extends to why information is important. Speculation is rarely seen at this level as the thinking is rule governed.	Speculation is apparent as you consider different arguments about what is important, what is happening and what is needed. The written account clearly exhibits discussion of why one option is better than another.	Interpretation involves the mixing of multiple sources of information, theory, research, experience and protocol. The review of information is conducted with regard to a clear purpose or goal. Speculation centres on what information can or should be used, as well as what is needed in the context explored.	Independent thinking involves adding information or ideas to a discussion that are entirely relevant but which many would not have considered. You question what is given, what is a problem or need, and what might represent a solution or opportunity. You speculate about what could be possible with reference to the highest standards of professional practice.
Making arguments	The arguments of others are put forward without question.	An array of arguments is presented, showing an awareness of options. The merits of different arguments are outlined. You determine which of the competing arguments is most credible.	Your own arguments are advanced with context, examining what is needed, ethical, relevant, realisable and coherent. Arguments may be combined from different places in order to build a convincing case for what can or should be done now.	Strikingly new arguments are presented, showing how you have thought about information in a fresh, new way. Arguments are cogent, coherently and compellingly made so that the reader feels they have learned something important.

Table 3.1 A framework of critical thinking

	Absolute thinking (early learning)	Transitional thinking	Contextual thinking	Independent thinking (advanced learning)
Spotting patterns	Information is randomly selected and arranged with no clear connections made between factors at play. Information may be recorded simply to fill spaces in the reflective framework or model used.	Information is linked one item to another, although why or how they relate to one another remains unclear in some instances. There is a notional understanding of cause and effect, and that sometimes things simply coexist and might be caused by something else that has gone before.	Now the items are discussed not only in relation to one another, but with regard to the context in which they arose. It is understood that some patterns hold good across settings (traits), but that context can also refine how something is viewed or experienced (states).	You recognise complex patterns of information that are shaped not only by context and trait behaviour, but which form wholes that can be described in conceptual terms (e.g. 'This is rehabilitation because it features these things'). These concepts can be used to recommend best fit nursing action.
Celebrating practice	The reasoning is trite. There is only one version of best practice, and why that has merit is not discussed.	Success is seen like the curate's egg – it is good in part. Focus shifts to what worked and why, but it is acknowledged that not all practice was perfect.	You examine why practice succeeded, with reference to the experience of different stakeholders.	The very way in which practice is conceived, what you and others are trying to do, becomes part of the discussion. Practice is understood in terms of values (your own and others), that which seems of the highest quality.
Correcting practice	Practice problems are not acknowledged; or if they are, they are ascribed to the behaviour of others alone.	Shortfalls and problems that lead to substandard practice are recognised, including your own. The reflection impresses as inquisitive and honest.	The reflection on shortfalls and problems is nuanced and relates directly to the issues that are of most concern in a given practice context. The work demonstrates how you think about what others hoped for and sets this against what they were trying to achieve.	Correcting practice involves a critical examination of beliefs, values and attitudes, the assumptions and philosophy that might shape care delivery. Independent thinkers are brave enough to explore these more fundamental issues as part of a practice review.

(Continued)

Table 3.2 (Continued)

	Absolute thinking (early learning)	Transitional thinking	Contextual thinking	Independent thinking (advanced learning)
Understanding self	There is little or no introspection; behaviour is often thought of as common sense.	You explore questions about why you thought or acted as you did, as well as the way this affects your approach to care.	The reasonableness of your approach in a given context is now honestly evaluated. You recognise that you have to understand how you negotiate care, as well as how that might or might not be suitable to the changing circumstances of healthcare.	Experience is understood as an opportunity to re-examine your own values, beliefs and attitudes. The account demonstrates the way that you interrogate how these relate to practice.
Understanding others	Others are understood in stereotypical terms and usually with reference to roles (e.g. 'Patients are like this, doctors are like that').	Others are understood as individuals, and usually with a history, background or training that helps to shape how they see practice. Individuals are respected for what they experience, do or achieve.	Others are understood as participants in a situation, each with their own perceptions and opinions relating to the care under way. The account is insightful and empathetic.	Others are perceived as individuals making sense of their existence, with their own philosophy and culture or traditions. The appropriateness of care is understood in terms of helping others to meet their personal needs.
Understanding profession and service	Profession and service are understood in stereotypical terms. You might 'label' what others do.	Profession and service are understood as complex, involving a lot of different contributions. Consideration shifts as to why the profession or service is as it is, as well as how and why it may be shifting.	Profession and service are understood as in transit, working with a society and patients whose needs are also changing. The fit might not be perfect, tensions are articulated, and you accept a shared responsibility in improving performance.	Healthcare service is understood as a negotiated process. Standards of practice as set by governing bodies must be understood and interpreted soundly in the face of changing healthcare demands. There is an imaginative and committed engagement in the best standards of care.

Table 3.2 A framework of reflection

Activity 3.2 Critical thinking

Select one of your previously marked essays now to re-examine it afresh against either Table 3.1 (if it was a theory essay) or Table 3.2 (if it was a reflective practice essay). You may or may not have welcomed your tutor's comments on the essay but the goal here is not to debate their assessment, it is to understand how your writing does or doesn't fit with different levels of reasoning. With reference to your chosen essay, and the assessment question set, identify the relevant critical or reflective thinking applications required there (e.g. asking questions, or understanding others). Against each of the relevant applications of critical thinking (column 1) place a pencil tick in the box which you think best represents the level of your reasoning in the essay concerned (columns 2–5). It's important to be honest when completing this exercise and to check your assessment with someone else. Where do you identify achievements in your essay and where does it seem lacking? If you're reviewing an essay from early in your course of studies, it's much less likely that you will have ticks in the far-right boxes–we progress over time.

As this answer is based on your own observation, there is no outline answer at the end of the chapter.

Discussing this exercise with your personal or module tutor is a valuable way to improve future written work. If you cannot discuss the essay with either of these, a review with a student companion might still be valuable. Remember, however, this exercise is completed only with an essay previously completed and marked. It is important not to collude on essay work currently in preparation, something that contravenes university study regulations. How uncomfortable or valuable was it to revisit an essay in this way? If you differed in your evaluation of the work, what were the key words, or applications of critical thinking that seemed more challenging to clarify? For example, was it hard to decide what in this instance represented a concept?

Preparing to write

Having explained different levels of reasoning and reflecting, we now turn to the business of preparing to write. Every time you prepare a piece of written work, you are selecting information to share, ways of expressing yourself which demonstrate that you have met the module learning outcomes and have made progress in your reasoning and reflecting. Students are surprised by the emphasis I place upon preparation time, imagining that we compose as we write. In my experience, there is real benefit in allocating 'thinking time' before you write. This is not simply a matter of making a plan; it is about distilling your thoughts before you try to use them to represent your learning. Tutors regularly comment that they can see in academic essays where students are thinking as they write. Problems include the following:

- not answering the question set;
- allocating the word count poorly (early sections getting the lion's share of words);
- material being presented in an incompletely reasoned state;
- essay conclusions falling short of requirements because students have never quite determined what they wish to finally claim;
- using others' work and representing it as your own (plagiarism is much more likely when you have allocated insufficient time to the preparation of work).

Activity 3.3   Critical thinking

I asked the case study students to each consider one of the preparations in Figure 3.1 that I think of as important in scholarly writing. Your challenge is to identify the opportunities you must engage in such preparatory work. What seemed most surprising or important to you here? How familiar or strange does this seem compared with your own usual essay preparation?

As this answer is based on your own observation, there is no outline answer at the end of the chapter.

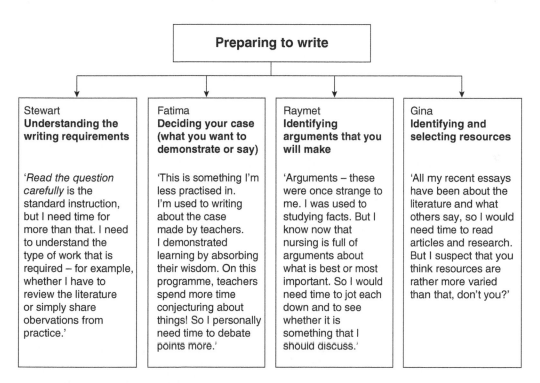

Figure 3.1   Preparing to write

Coming from a different professional background, Stewart is already attuned to the need to understand the writing task set. Nursing courses include a wide variety of forms of writing. For example, if you are asked to present a case study, you will need to write reflectively but you will also need to include elements of strategy linked to care. I suggest not only that you read the requirements carefully (the assignment brief) but also that you take time to clarify any concerns and queries with the person who set the brief. Pay particular attention to the wording of assessment questions. Does the assignment brief indicate what is really required by 'critically discuss', for instance? If you fail to clarify such matters and guess the requirements, mistakes can prove costly in terms of grades achieved.

Many of you may empathise with Fatima's response about the difficulty of adopting a position within a piece of coursework. In the past, students have often been required to summarise what others have said, especially teachers. Looking back to Table 3.1 and its points on making arguments, you can see that this represents absolute thinking, and something more is typically required in an undergraduate module. Past courses may have been more pedagogical, requiring you simply to replicate others' teaching. The move from a background where you are required to demonstrate what has been taught to you to one where you must reason more for yourself is difficult for students (Magnusson and Zackariasson, 2018; Bagnasco et al., 2020). In my experience, this is heightened where students are required to 'take a stance on an issue' of their own. For example, in rehabilitation, where work is shared with patients and lay carers, you might be asked to state what represents a reasonable level of input from those that we care for. What do you expect patients and their relatives to learn and do, and what do you think nurses should contribute? In these and similar matters, you do need to make a case, and it is important for you to be completely clear about this before you start.

In Figure 3.1, Raymet's points are important: students often wonder when an argument becomes a fact. Moreover, if you are to grapple with a series of arguments, how should they best be arranged?

In nursing courses, it is often necessary to present a series of arguments, each of which supports the case or position that we adopt. You will often find within UK universities that the case or position is conventionally stated early within the academic paper, with the main text then used to rehearse arguments and counterarguments, which help the student to sum up insights within their conclusion. There are other approaches within reflective writing, which I explore in Part 3. Such essays are typical of what tests transitional or contextual thinking (see Table 3.1). For example, your case or position may be that nurses should educate patients to take on self-care activities. Arguments in support of this include: (a) patients gain independence through their own learning; (b) it is not economically viable to go on delivering all the care, so patients and relatives need to develop their own skills; and (c) patients develop greater self-esteem through the process of learning to care for themselves. This may or may not be your experience of previous learning, where perhaps you revealed your position incrementally at the end of your paper. However, the case-first sequence is the reasoning norm for more philosophical essays within nursing, so if you have difficulties making that transition, it is worth discussing the adjustments you are trying to make with your personal tutor.

Let's summarise that important point with an illustration. My case is that rehabilitation is collaborative; I cannot require the patient to make progress, cannot assure success unless they are engaged in the process too. I write that in my essay, as part of the introduction. Afterwards I rehearse what supports or counters my case. For example, patients' motivation and learning ability varies widely. But I might note that incremental achievement is a key motivator for patients. The more they learn and sense progress the more they are motivated to improve again. This sounds familiar, doesn't it? It's the arrangement of argument and premises you read about in Chapter 1, only now we have taken it up to a new level, using the same principles for your essay, as a whole.

Gina is correct that tutors envisage students using a variety of resources as part of their academic writing, and that it takes time to select what will be included in a piece of coursework. Observations from practice, arguments articulated by others in interview, and hospital care philosophies are just a few of the things that could support what you write about. It takes time to evaluate each of these and judge how each resource will be linked to the arguments made (e.g. 'This supports my argument, that reminds us that there are alternative perspectives'). We could hope that there is a definitive list of resources to be drawn upon, but I'm afraid that this is rarely the case. You will need to judge what is most pertinent. Tutors often signal what they value strongly, for instance, research evidence versus the results of patient experience audits. The astute student notes such things as well as exploring what they believe themselves.

Avoiding plagiarism

Plagiarism is the use of other people's written work, figures, tables or diagrams, and the representation of these as your own work within an academic paper (Mbutho and Hutchings, 2021; Price, 2014). Plagiarism carries severe penalties at university. At the least, you may receive a written warning; at worst, you may have an academic paper failed or you could be dismissed from the course altogether. It is therefore vital to prepare for writing in ways that limit the risk of committing plagiarism. Each of the following represents good preparation:

- Read very carefully the university rules and regulations regarding the correct representation of the work of others within your academic essays. This can usually be found within the course handbook or the study skills section of the course web page. Make a point of asking your tutors about anything that you do not understand.
- Use a notebook to record all the sources of information that you have used, including websites. Do this immediately when you find helpful material. Make a note of the website address (its URL) so that you can find it again. One of the temptations is to use notes made from websites, and then – because you cannot find the reference details later – to represent the words used as your own.
- Do not assume that because there is no author's name evident on a web page, it does not need to be referenced. The default position should be that where author

details seem to be missing, you should treat the organisation that runs the web page as the author of the work.

- Get into the habit of using quotation marks regularly at the start and end of a passage of copied words. If you paraphrase work (i.e. rephrase the points in your own words), make sure that you do a thorough job. Changing just the odd word within the sentence does not constitute paraphrasing, and you may be told that you have plagiarised the work. Imagine that the original text that you read said this: 'Rehabilitation is both an educational and a support process, one in which the patient is required to actively engage and one which requires the nurse to strategise, evaluating how well the patient is doing.' You might paraphrase this as: 'Nurses work strategically with patients, teaching and supporting them, adjusting rehabilitation work as they go.' The paraphrase captures the essence of what has been written without using the same words. You still then need to acknowledge the source, indicating the author's name and year of publication within brackets in the text.

- Reserve enough thinking time before you write. However daunting it seems, you do have to decide what you think about others' reported work. Examiners respect that your points will not always seem profound, but they do need to understand what sense you make of that which has been reviewed.

- Do not share essay drafts or past assignment answers with other students. There is a risk that others may copy your work and you could be charged with aiding and abetting them (academic collusion). Universities use software that can show the similarities between student work received, including that which was submitted in the past.

- Do not be tempted to purchase essay work from the internet. Not only is this considered a calculated effort to cheat (one mandating a severe penalty), but you may also be using something that is in any case not fit for purpose. Tutors are keenly aware of what you have written in the past and what this essay requires, so subterfuge essays are often spotted.

- Check to see whether your university offers you access to a script-checking service such as Turnitin (www.turnitin.com). Turnitin compares passages of your own work against that which exists within other published and website work, showing you where your words match those elsewhere. There is no problem with found matches where you have attributed the source of the material and used quotation marks appropriately; but where sentences or longer passages of your work match those from elsewhere and no attribution is recorded, vital corrections need to be made.

The basics of structure

Pieces of academic work have a beginning, a middle and an end, and must seem complete and coherent. It is this quality of completeness and coherence, together with authority, clarity and precision, that we search for when planning a paper. Completeness and coherence are supported by the way in which we structure the written work; authority is determined by how we present and support arguments; and clarity and precision are affected by how we help others to navigate the paper, as well as through the way in which we decide what to include and what to leave out. If we force too much information into an essay, clarity suffers.

Activity 3.4   Research

To help you explore structure more fully, select an article published within a nursing journal and read through it, noting how it is structured. Pay particular attention to the way that sections are set out and what sorts of things are discussed in each section. While published works are more polished than those submitted for coursework assessment, they nevertheless include relevant structural features that we can discuss.

When you have finished reading your chosen article, answer my questions at the end of each of the following sections.

As this answer is based on your chosen article, there is no outline answer at the end of the chapter.

Introducing the work

All pieces of academic work need an introduction, which has four roles:

* to identify the subject matter of the written piece;
* to secure the reader's attention and interest;
* to establish the writer's position or perspective;
* to set any contexts within which the paper needs to be understood.

It is possible to establish the subject matter by stating the essay question set or to simply say at the outset, for example, 'This essay is written about the rehabilitation work of the nurse.' However, there are slightly more adventurous ways of introducing a subject. An academic essay is not journalism, but like journalists we are required to interest our readers in the essay's subject matter, even if they are examiners and are being paid to read our work. We need a 'hook' to encourage them to read on. Two common ways of doing this are:

* Start with a bold point that highlights the importance of the subject matter (e.g. 'There is at least anecdotal evidence that nurses and patients are not always working to the same ends during rehabilitation').
* Introduce a dilemma that needs to be addressed (e.g. 'There is a problem with patient rehabilitation, and this is linked to what we consider ideal and what seems possible given resource constraints').

You will need to decide whether your introduction will be presented in the first person singular (referring to 'I') or in the third person, referring to 'the nurse' or 'nurses'.

First-person singular is the norm where any form of reflective writing is required. Whereas in the third person you refer to 'the author', it is important to be aware of literature review traps – are you referring to the author of other papers reviewed or to you, the author of this essay?

If your work concerns practice or an area of professional discourse (e.g. applied science, pharmacology), your introduction needs to make this clear. You might, for instance, refer to a client group to whom your work concerns (e.g. post-operative patients) or a particular area of practice (e.g. the use of analgesia).

Activity 3.5   Reflection

Examine your chosen article to establish whether the introduction achieves all the aims of an introduction, as listed above. If any of the key features are missing, what are the implications for the rest of the piece? Look back to Table 3.1 to examine what the introduction offers as regards levels of critical thinking. Can you see how setting out a case early on, focusing the essay, might help you to demonstrate clear arguments and show how you are interpreting a subject?

As this answer is based on your own observation, there is no outline answer at the end of the chapter.

Signposting the work

Towards the end of the introduction to your work, you need to help the reader understand how the rest of the work is set out (e.g. 'This essay is set out in the following sections ...'). Signposting is not only a description of the rest of the work, though; it frequently includes an indication of the stance that you take and the purpose of your paper. You may indicate, for instance, that this paper on rehabilitation nursing considers the role of the nurse in section 1 and the role of patients and lay carers in section 2, and then debates the liaison work between the two groups in section 3 (e.g. 'The paper makes the case that rehabilitation is a negotiated activity and one that requires careful liaison between stakeholders').

Activity 3.6   Critical thinking

Did you spot signposting in the work that you chose to read? It frequently consists of just one very important paragraph at the end of the introduction. Does the signposting within your reviewed work help you to read forward with a clear purpose, knowing what the author is trying to do?

As this answer is based on your own observation, there is no outline answer at the end of the chapter.

Developing the main body of the work

Classically, academic essays include a main text with few subsections, and they rarely include figures or tables. Within nursing, however, the conventions are rapidly changing, and it is usual to arrange the work using subheadings to help the reader navigate your work, as well as including both figures and tables where these help you to make a point quickly and clearly. Check your course handbook to establish the local norms. My own preference is to encourage writing that helps the reader to follow your arguments and includes features that are similar to those used when writing for publication (e.g. section headings, figures and/or tables).

What remains important in academic papers is that you write in disciplined paragraphs, with short sentences that enable you to make clear points. Where you do use figures, tables or appendices, they must all be clearly referred to in the text and within brackets (e.g. 'see Figure 1', 'Table 3 refers to …').

What do I mean by a disciplined paragraph? In practical terms:

- It attends to a single subject (e.g. ascertaining the patient's readiness to rehabilitate).
- It includes clear points and your own or others' arguments (e.g. 'While economic pressures exist to speed up rehabilitation, the readiness of a patient to learn skills still affects the pace of their progress').
- It provides support for what has been stated. This is often where references to the literature come in, but – as we have noted – other evidence gleaned from practice could be referred to (e.g. 'An example patient helps to make the case. Mr X reported that he felt paralysed by fear regarding taking exercise after his heart attack. He worried that staff had not completely understood the risks.').

Sentences that extend beyond a couple of lines of text are much more likely to seem ambiguous to the reader. Being scholarly does not necessarily mean writing longer sentences or cramming more information into a paragraph.

The last key consideration regarding the main text is that you build a series of arguments. To demonstrate that you are thinking critically, it is important not to accept points at face value. For this reason, a paragraph that makes one argument could, in some instances, be followed by another paragraph that makes a second argument. But it is important by the end of your work to demonstrate that you have reached your own conclusions, even if this is only to suggest that the debate continues. Remember that in transitional and contextual reasoning, you will have to demonstrate possible arguments and review their merits. You will need to determine the best fit arguments to a context of interest, whether that be clinical practice or perhaps a review of nursing theories and their ease of use. So, turning once more to our example, we might spend one paragraph arguing the above point about the importance of patients' readiness to commence rehabilitation and then add a second paragraph which reminds the reader that prolonged inactivity increases the risk of post-myocardial infarction complications.

On balance, then, the recommended way forward is physical rehabilitation and consistent psychological support while patients test their limits.

Activity 3.7   Critical thinking

Examine your chosen article to identify some examples of what you think are especially successful paragraphs and to list the arguments you can see being developed within the main text of the paper. How does this structure compare with some of your own past essays? Can you see how the work starts to have a bigger impact because of its structure?

As this answer is based on your own observation, there is no outline answer at the end of the chapter.

Reaching a conclusion

Academic coursework (unless otherwise instructed) requires a conclusion. Within the conclusion, there should be no substantial new material. Its purpose is to sum up what has been written so far. However, the essay must show what sense has been made about the arguments presented. Beyond all those points about helping the patient rehabilitate, what does this amount to? The author needs to deduce what the arguments support. Perhaps it is first to support patients because they are doing a lot of the rehabilitation work. Perhaps it is to co-ordinate rehabilitation work. Perhaps it is that if physiotherapy is given before patient education has been delivered, patient anxiety might be increased.

I discussed conclusions with Gina, and she likened them to the point where you must tie off a balloon having inflated it fully. Essays are inflated with evidence and arguments, but if at the end you simply signal you don't know what this all amounts to, then you have not tied off the metaphorical balloon.

Activity 3.8   Critical thinking

Scrutinise your chosen paper to see whether the conclusion achieves the above. Do not be surprised if you identify some shortfalls here – even published papers sometimes include weak conclusions. Did the conclusion make reference to a case that was stated at the start of the essay or article?

As this answer is based on your own observation, there is no outline answer at the end of the chapter.

Adopting the right voice

We come at last to the business of 'voice'. You might be surprised that I use a term more associated with singing to describe scholarly writing. By voice, I mean conveying your thoughts in such a way that your thinking is demonstrated as something that seems orderly, measured, critical or reflective, as the need dictates. Academic voice helps you to portray that you are thinking at a higher level of critical thinking. Singers use a voice to convey emotions or drama. Students need, through their texts, to use a voice to illustrate or represent their learning. We have already conveyed two ways in which your work will seem more scholarly: first, developing a coherent structure for your work; and second, building a series of arguments that demonstrate your reasoning. There remain, though, some important niceties in the ways in which you write (i.e. use your voice) that will enhance your reputation as a scholar.

Activity 3.9   Critical thinking

Look at some sample sentences that the four case study student nurses used in their earliest essays. They are at pains to remind us that their work has improved since. There are some classic faults within these short extracts that demonstrate less than scholarly work, and I invite you to identify them.

Gina: That patients wait, lying on trolleys within a corridor or a corner of casualty, is utterly appalling.

Stewart: Time is money, so the doctor's stay at the bedside is always short and patients ask others what has then been decided as regards their treatment.

Raymet: The assessment I made of the patient was holistic. I examined their rash and listened carefully to their anxieties.

Fatima: A tutor has explained that patients sometimes only want to please the nurse, rather than state their real concerns. This seems right to me.

My answers to this activity are included in the text below.

Did you spot the fact that in Activity 3.9, Gina was using hyperbole (i.e. accentuating a point made in a heavy-handed or excessive way)? While we might share dismay at the length of time patients wait to secure a bed, and would not commend long waiting times, the conventions of academic writing are that we express opinion in rather more measured terms. In this example, a more measured critique of this situation might be to observe that the lengthy waits were undignified and that they raised questions about service standards. The phrase 'utterly appalling' appeals to the emotions of the reader rather than their intellect, and we do not convey analysis so clearly. A scholarly voice is measured and resists hyperbole. For example, when evaluating practice, 'the care had specific benefits', not 'the care was simply fantastic'.

Stewart's fault in this example concerned what we call a colloquialism (i.e. a form of shorthand writing that we assume the reader understands). 'Time is money' is a well-known aphorism that describes how people prioritise their time using economic considerations. But used in this context, it hardly does justice to the doctor. Colloquial language often conveys the sort of absolute thinking seen in Tables 3.1 and 3.2.

The fault in Raymet's writing is rather more subtle but is nonetheless a good example of where the academic voice has not yet been developed. If work is to be precise, it is necessary to use terms and concepts with care. In this instance, Raymet is referring to holism and claiming that the assessment of a patient was holistic. However, 'holistic' refers to four major aspects of a person's life and experience: the physical, psychological, social and spiritual. It suggests that the care delivered engages deeply and comprehensively with the patient's experience (George et al., 2017). What Raymet reports here is not a holistic assessment of the patient, but one that concentrates upon the patient's rash (physical) and anxieties (psychological). Checking a dictionary can help to resolve this issue.

There are two possible problems with the academic voice in Fatima's extract. First, there are usually conventions associated with the referencing of sources, and here Fatima is not following them. If she has been encouraged to include personal discourses with a tutor within academic work, it is necessary to state in brackets the nature of that (e.g. 'personal e-mail communication with tutor X'). Second, students sometimes present work that is designed to please the marker of the finished work. They may refer with approval to what the examiner has taught, said or written elsewhere. In scholarly writing, though, examiners wish to learn what the student has reasoned rather than what the tutor has taught. It is necessary to demonstrate your own judgement and evaluation of issues rather than to simply approve those that you think might please someone else.

Thus, a scholarly voice is one that:

- acknowledges the source of points and perspectives of others (in the literature or elsewhere);
- demonstrates your own reasoning and reflection;
- uses terms precisely and consistently;
- expresses points in a measured rather than emotive way;
- avoids forms of shorthand reasoning such as colloquialisms.

Chapter summary

I return to the matter of scholarly writing again in Part 3. It is important here, however, to acknowledge the above precepts of good writing, some of which can seem implicit rather than explained within the course that you study. Pausing to consider what is required of you by your tutor and the university, as well as where that fits and does not fit with what you have learned before, can help you to understand what seems more challenging about study. Most of what is required is determined by the need to convey your learning in as clear and accessible a manner as possible: by adhering to simple practices, by writing a paper that has a clear beginning, middle and end, and by signposting the reader through the work. It is about considering how much information you can or should include within a sentence or paragraph, as well as whether your work within that paragraph has strayed away from its subject. It is certainly about good spelling and grammar, as well as checking work before it is submitted.

Of all the fundamental errors in scholarly writing that I see within nurse education programmes, there are three which recur frequently. Some students fail to appreciate what sort of writing they are asked to provide. Like Stewart, they need to clarify the requirements set, usually by taking questions to the tutor. Other students begin to write long before they have concluded what they think. Tables 3.1 and 3.2 emphasise just how important and complex thinking can be. Students are then hard-pressed to identify what case they wish to present. 'Thinking time' is more important than 'writing time' and it is worth investing in, especially if you jot down notes about your developing ideas. A third group of students rush forward with their writing, failing to attend to the academic voice required within assignments and using imprecise terms. The net effect is that their work seems ill-considered and hurriedly prepared.

Many of the papers that students have criticised as 'too descriptive' are associated with such faults. Arguments are lacking and the ideas discussed have been handled in a shorthand way.

Examining examples of scholarly writing in different places will help you to identify what conveys learning clearly and well. By studying the resources that you find within the university library, you will be much better placed to represent your reasoning and reflection when it comes to work that carries course marks.

Further reading

Greetham, B (2018) *How to write better essays*, 4th edition. London: Palgrave Macmillan.

This is an accessible and logical guide to the business of finding information and making coherent notes, as well as turning these into coherent and adequately source-cited essays.

Matthews, J (2020) *How to write an awesome paragraph: step by step* (independently published via Amazon UK).

This short (93-page) basic text is worth dipping into if you have the gravest doubts about your ability to write in an academic manner. It goes straight to the heart of what is structurally required, writing coherent and convincing paragraphs. The examples used are not from nursing, but if you are getting lots of critical commentary about your ability to structure an argument, this might be one source to return to.

Price, B (2017) How to write a reflective practice case study. *Primary Healthcare*, 27(9): 35–42.

There is a paucity of guidance on how to write well by combining both experience and evidence together. This article explains how to structure a piece of writing clearly, establishing why the topic is important for your readership.

Wallace, M and Wray, A (2021) *Critical reading and writing for postgraduates,* 4th edition. London: Sage.

While my own text reviews valuable principles for critical thinking, reflection and writing across academic levels, I think that this text adds something more, for example as regards the preparation of dissertations. It's not specifically focused on healthcare, but the guidance holds good in most instances.

Useful website

Each university produces its own guide to good academic writing processes and sets out requirements for the way in which assignments should be presented. Conventions may differ by university. I therefore direct you to the study skills section of your university website rather than prompting you to a wider trawl of the internet.

Part 2

Critical thinking and reflecting in nursing contexts

Chapter 4   Making sense of lectures

NMC Future Nurse: Standards of Proficiency for Registered Nurses

Because the subject matter of lectures varies widely, there are no specific standards to link to. The skills covered in this chapter underpin how you successfully learn and achieve all of the standards within the environment of lectures.

Chapter aims

After reading this chapter, you will be able to:

- detail ways to engage with a lecture so as to enhance the quality of your learning;
- summarise ways in which to prepare for a lecture;
- explain why questions are so important to learning in a lecture;
- summarise important things to do after a lecture has ended.

Introduction

When I asked my case study students about the importance of lectures within their course, they reported several things. First, lectures were seen as the key teaching component of the course. While distance learning course students measured courses by teaching materials delivered (in print or online), in-attendance course students rated courses on the number and the quality of lectures provided (see Gross et al., 2015 and Feistauer and Richter, 2017 for a wider debate on student evaluations of lectures). Gina observed that students expected instruction on the subject matter of the course. While there were other communal and tutor-facilitated campus-based ways to learn, perhaps some that exercised critical thinking even more strongly (e.g. seminars discussing selected literature), the lecture was often the students' foci when evaluating a course. The second thing that they noted was that lectures were now strongly influenced by technology. A lecture might be recorded and offered via the course website (Wolf, 2018). This afforded opportunities to view it at leisure and to return to it again and again to augment note-taking. If a lecture was very instructional (Gina cited the example of physiology) then a recorded lecture could be revisited several times to understand the important processes discussed.

Fatima observed that the quality of lectures might vary markedly. Where a researcher was invited to lecture it was not automatic that they always explained matters clearly. There was a risk that experts could overestimate students' reasoning, either proceeding too quickly or guessing inaccurately what students already understood. Fatima acknowledged that some lectures were 'brilliant', but this was usually because the lecturer started with a sound appreciation of what worried students most. A good lecturer was usually 'passionate about teaching'. When evaluating lectures, it was important to be offered focused critique about what had been difficult. Were concepts left unexplained? Did the lecture try to cover too much information, racing through material which was new to the students? How were questions handled and when were they scheduled? Detailed and measured critique was more likely to improve lectures in the future.

Your course is likely to present you with an array of lectures. Some will be delivered in real time (with opportunities for a question-and-answer session). Some will be recorded either as a video or a podcast (sound recording). The lectures will operate to different purpose as illustrated in Table 4.1. Appreciating just what the lecture is designed to do will help you to manage your expectations and to extract the best learning from it.

Activity 4.1   Reflection

Recall now two or three successful lectures that you enjoyed. Identify what seemed to make the lecture such a success. What was the purpose of the lectures, and did that seem to affect what you took away from it (see Table 4.1)? If you preferred just one kind of lecture, does that suggest anything problematic about your expectations of learning on the course? If so, it may be important to discuss this with your personal tutor. Did you contribute to the lecture in some way, for example by asking questions?

As this answer is based on your own observation, there is no outline answer at the end of the chapter.

Preparing for the lecture

Raymet and I talked about difficulties that she had encountered with lectures on her course, and we analysed what resolved those later. The first thing she remembered

Purpose	Explanatory notes
To instruct or explain e.g. lectures on the physiology of homeostasis (Chirillo et al., 2021)	These can work well in 'real time' and recorded presentations. If there has been a series of such instructional lectures check whether these are supported with a tutorial where you can take stock of what has been taught. It's a good idea to match instructional lectures with relevant chapters in your textbooks, either as part of preparation for the lecture or review afterwards.
To demonstrate e.g. How to conduct a patient-history-taking session. The lecturer might deploy video clips or volunteer patients.	Practical demonstrations take place either in the clinical area or within a skills laboratory. Confident lecturers may though run a best principles demonstration before an assembled lecture room audience, and this works very well if you are able to witness a dialogue. You should expect that the lecture will have break points where the lecturer (and perhaps the co-presenter) pause to invite discussion of what you have witnessed. Attend to both what was discussed, and the communication techniques used.
To illustrate critical thinking and reflection (JuHee et al., 2016) e.g. the lecturer 'thinks aloud' work involved in negotiating care with patients.	These are among the most valuable lectures of all. First, the lecturer acknowledges the uncertainty of practice, the exploratory and problem-solving nature of the nurse's work. Second, they share with you something of their philosophy and values, both influential in the design of care. You learn how they enquire and deliberate. A consummate performer of this kind of lecture shares with you the humility of enquiry and can reassure you that critical thinking process improves with practice. Theory, philosophy, research evidence and practical utility within the care setting are all combined.
To map the complexity of nursing practice e.g. the lecturer rehearses the ways in which different ethical principles might compete when examining care (Skirbekk et al., 2018).	Nurses confront complex and untidy clinical situations. Admitted to an exploration of this kind, it becomes easier for you to understand why trite, absolute interpretations of care are so often inadequate. A well-designed lecture though will offer you hope, sharing principles that can reduce the uncertainty faced. Sometimes these lectures take the form of a guided literature review.
To excite and motivate you e.g. inspirational teachers are invited to recount the ways in which they have conceived care.	I have been inspired by many speakers, those who seem to excel in care and to exemplify creative thinking. Beware though being swept up by idealism, questions about what doesn't work so well, and what remains a challenge, are still important.

Table 4.1 Example purposes of the lecture

was how she saw the lectures as one-off events. Each module was populated with what seemed a range of loosely related lectures. A mix of speakers meant it was harder to see the design of the series. The second thing she reflected was that she approached the lecture thinking that learning began with the lecture. The lectures delivered 'truth', and then it was her job to absorb that afterwards.

Framing

What later helped Raymet and might help you is the reminder that we do the learning and that the lecture provides information or a skill to assist with that. We must frame the lecture in the context of our own learning to date and what the module learning objectives or outcomes state that we must work towards. Course designers think of this process as sandwich learning, as students go back and forth between module content (that taught) and their own personal processing of information received (that learned) (Bock et al., 2020). So, what do we mean when we frame a lecture? Framing entails the following:

- refreshing your memory of the module focus, what is covered and what you are meant to achieve (learning work);
- anticipating the topic of the lecture and writing down any experiences or questions, perhaps values or beliefs that seem important to you there (learning journey);
- acknowledging any doubts about what you currently understand (learning hurdles);
- exploring a trusted textbook or recommended articles that introduce the topic to you (learning resource).

Well-designed module handbooks will commend preparatory reading for a course of lectures ahead (Hernandez-Acevedo et al., 2022). The reading is carefully selected to introduce you to new ideas that the lecturers refer to. Raymet explained that lectures seemed like seeds planted into soil. New material must work with (but not necessarily confirm) experience and learning to date (that already planted). We take the material and try to evaluate it. Raymet didn't initially believe that she was permitted opening values about healthcare. Legitimate values came fresh from the lecturer. 'I thought of myself like a blank slate,' she told me, 'so I thought I was slow understanding what lecturers taught. I didn't realise that some of what they said questioned my existing values. I didn't appreciate that lectures challenged what I already believed. So, learning might involve adding things but also discarding or adjusting other things.'

Framing offers a chance to understand what you think and feel before the lecture is met with. It can help you to understand how knowledge is expanding and becoming more nuanced and how it might challenge you. Learning engages our emotions as well as our intellect so framing a forthcoming lecture with reading and reflection is a very good thing to do. If you frame for the lecture well, then you might ask much more searching questions later and secure bigger insights than if you came cold to the lecture room.

To help you frame forthcoming lectures here are a series of questions that might assist (my four Cs).

Context

What is the context of this lecture and why is it important? Imagine a lecture delivered on cross-infection control and hygiene. That becomes more important in the light of the Covid-19 pandemic (Cui et al., 2019). But it may be personally important to you as you reflect on practices observed in the clinical area. Were protocols clear? Was there more than one way to practise safely within such protocols?

Connections

What seems to connect with the anticipated subject matter of this coming lecture? Lectures often operate in family groups, as it were. A lecture on ethical theory relates closely to professionalism. They are in a subject matter family of professional etiquette. Ethics highlight professional responsibilities but also raises some challenges as regards practising well. Ethical responsibilities (patients' rights) may compete with one another (Sokol, 2018).

Causes and consequences

How do you think the lecturer will treat causes and consequences in this lecture? In nursing, both are vitally important. Much of our time is spent trying to understand causes and to anticipate – and in some instances avert – consequences. Most lectures have something to say about causes and consequences, even when they are not about diseases and healthcare problems. For instance, if you attend a lecture on the pharmacology of analgesics then a question might quickly arise, what happens when these drugs are taken with other kinds by perhaps an elderly patient? Causes and consequences remind us of the need to think about caveats and precautions and they can remind the lecturer that thinking solely within one subject silo might not assist the learner that much.

Caring

Nursing is fundamentally about caring in a professional, effective and efficient way (Ellis et al., 2020). So, what might the anticipated subject matter of this lecture mean for caring? Let us imagine a lecture on psychoses and the ways in which these alter the perceptions of patients. What might it be like to deliver emotional support to a psychotically ill patient who suffers from delusions or hallucinations? Anticipating the care implications of a lecture is a good way of piquing interest in subject matter.

Activity 4.2   Reflection

Think now of a lecture that seemed controversial to you now. Why did it seem challenging? What should follow next? Should you challenge your existing values and beliefs revising some of them? Should you consult others the better to understand the discrepancy felt? Would framing have helped you with this? My reflections appear at the end of the chapter.

Engaging with the real-time lecture

It is now time to consider how we can usefully engage effectively with the lecturer in a real-time lecture. Engagement here refers to three key activities. First, showing the lecturer that you are attending to what they are sharing (Ko et al., 2019). Lecturers depend on the visual cues that you share through your facial expressions. Just how far – and how fast – they progress with their points depends on you honouring them with an attentive gaze. Do not worry if you frown – all information of this kind signals something useful to the lecturer.

The second activity relates to the questions that you and your peers ask. While a lecturer may have an agenda as regards what they wish to convey within the time available, no thoughtful teacher rejects sincere questions. Your learning is at least as important as their exposition, but you will need to agree with your lecturer the best times to ask questions. In explanatory lectures (Table 4.1), lecturers typically need to convey a chunk of information, that which they anticipate will help you understand the subject better. They may wish to take questions at the end of the session. Often, however, question opportunities are punctuated at key points within the lecture. This is particularly important where the lecturer builds an idea for you to study (critical thinking illustration, Table 4.1). You are asked to consider a series of arguments that add up to something bigger. You are theorising with the lecturer. Forming those theories, and perhaps even reaching a template for practice, however, is only possible if you check your understanding en route.

The third activity is responding to the lecturer's own challenges. Classically, these are posed in the form of questions that the lecturer invites the audience to offer answers to. But some lecturers are yet more skilful, and they set up provocative statements, those that you are invited to debate (Wolff et al., 2015). Of course, if you are sitting with your head down making notes, some of those may pass you by. The lecturer may want to dissuade you from simply accepting the arguments of others without question. So, listen carefully for any seemingly provocative arguments that the lecturer might offer up to you.

Discussion with your lecturer, as well as possibly with other students, deepens your understanding of key issues. It may certainly help you to remember points that could be raised later in a piece of coursework. It is in teaching sessions such as lectures that you learn to enquire, and in some measure – depending on the format of the lecture – to question and debate. Remember that, in Table 3.1, higher levels of critical thinking are associated with asking how arguments fit with contexts. So, asking questions about whether the espoused ideas work in practice is extremely important. It is necessary to ask yourself, and perhaps the lecturers too, what conditions would have to prevail before an argument made were true. Imagine that your lecturer was sharing with you some of the rights that they believe underpin nursing care. The patient has a right to confidentiality, but you remember that care is often delivered in communal environments where medical rounds are completed. So, a question about possible challenges and compromises to the right of confidentiality is entirely reasonable: 'I noted your points about confidentiality, but what about medical rounds and the discussion of problems at the bedside? Is this a problem?'

We need to ruminate on what has been said by the lecturer. If you are ready to explore how the claims made by the lecturer affect your current values, beliefs and attitudes, you are beginning to engage with the highest possible level of reflective thinking, described in Table 3.2 (page 51).

Activity 4.3   Reflection

Look now at your notebook to see how you arrange notes in lecture sessions. What gets recorded there and then, and what (if anything) is written up later? How extensive are your lecture session notes? Thinking back to Chapter 1, as well as what you have already read about theorising and the discovery of templates, what advantages can you see in building notes after the lecture has finished? We will turn to note-taking shortly, but for now I encourage you to examine what you do already.

As this answer is based on your own observation, there is no outline answer at the end of the chapter.

Listening and making notes

It is important to trust your memory as you engage with the lecture. Let me explain what I mean by that. A common student concern in lectures is to record as much information as possible because you fear that you will otherwise forget everything: 'If I could but note more information down, later I would write the perfect essay!' In practice, though, if your notes from the lecture are chock-full of quotes, facts and theories, it is likely that you may have missed many of the connecting ideas which the lecturer shared. For example, why is cancer staging so important? How does the nurse gather together information to help the patient cope with what cancer staging reveals? The questions of 'why' and 'how' are more difficult to capture when you are making real-time notes in the lecture. It requires so many more words to adequately record, and in the meantime the lecture has moved on. For that reason, it is important to polish your notes (i.e. turn them into sentences and paragraphs, fuller bullet points) after the lecture, and in the meantime listen more to what the lecturer is saying.

This raises the question of what your notes should look like as they leave the lecture room (see Activity 4.3). Because learning is also a personal matter, I do not wish to be didactic about how to take notes in a lecture. I do, however, want to recommend a basic drafting layout for the note-taking page that aids critical thinking afterwards. The trick is to capture enough notes to enable you to write a fuller summary after the lecture.

Start by dividing each blank page of your notes into three columns. If it helps, work with the pages in landscape rather than portrait format. The left-hand column should be a relatively narrow one, perhaps just 20 per cent of the page width. Label this 'lecture link'. It is simply going to be the place where you note the slide or screen that the notes relate to. Having this link to your lecture and handout will enable you to connect your thinking accurately to the points made by the lecturer. So, perhaps in this column I might record 'slide 1: role of cancer staging'. This is the title of the slide that the lecturer shared, and it is probably also the title used for the same section of the lecture handout. If you are permitted to audio-record the lecture, then it might also refer to the recording point where important arguments were made.

I suggest that you label the middle column of the page 'themes'. It is here that you will jot down your ideas, questions and pivotal points that seem to relate closely to the stage of the lecture that you have recorded in the left-hand column. In this area, you are going to jot down your thoughts – it is not a space to try to recreate the lecturer's slide or handout. The urge to try to reproduce all that the lecturer presents is a very human one, but try to resist it. Negotiate the supply of regular handouts and trust your notes as a place to think on paper. This column should occupy around 60 per cent of the width of your page. Perhaps here I might write things such as 'Staging indicates disease progression', 'Late stage equals disease spread/poorer prognosis', 'But staging different for different cancers', 'Wow, how to explain this to the patient?' and 'Does staging change if treatment successful?' Do you see how it comprises just snippet information and questions? It includes my emotional responses too (e.g. 'wow'). These become your prompts for fuller notes after the lecture has finished. Remember that the proportion of time spent in lectures at university is relatively small – more time should indeed be dedicated to note development.

I suggest that you label the right-hand column of the page 'keywords/references' (around 20 per cent of page width). If the lecturer does not provide a handout, then you will need a space to copy down any pivotal references that you should follow up later. You will need to explore keywords in the library to deepen your command of the ideas shared. A keyword (or phrase) in the example lecture that I am using might be 'distal spread'. This refers to the existence of tumour cells in a new area of the body, perhaps the other side of the mediastinum. Distal spread is important because it affects available treatment modalities.

Activity 4.4   Critical thinking

Look back now at your reflections in Activity 4.3 and determine whether the idea of a structured note page linked to lecture handouts helps you. Does it help you to order your notes and facilitate revision for coursework assignments or examinations? If these notes need polishing in a subsequent write-up, how do you think this might benefit the development of your critical thinking?

I offer some of my own suggestions at the end of the chapter.

The use of questions to facilitate learning

Questions feature regularly within lectures, and many students worry about these. They fear that a question posed by the tutor will seem difficult, and that not venturing an answer or offering the wrong answer might tarnish their reputation. You will only develop your critical-thinking abilities, however, if you are prepared to engage in questions, both asking your own and answering those of your tutor. Questions enable you to fill in gaps in your knowledge and ascertain whether your current grasp of a subject is complete. Tutors know that it feels daunting for a student to engage in questioning, so they use a technique that allows the more confident students to venture answers to questions first. As you attend your next lecture, notice how the tutor poses a question first to the whole group, inviting possible answers from students. The tutor 'poses' the question, then 'pauses', allowing time for everyone to give the question due consideration, and then 'pounces' (Jones, 2018). If 'pounce' sounds rather intimidating, remember that pose/pause/pounce is simply an aide-memoire for teachers learning their craft. The 'pounce' usually involves inviting a student who has signalled an interest in answering to share their thoughts. Tutors are taught *not* to embarrass individual students in the class. Where your answer is incomplete, you will usually be congratulated on the successful part of the answer before the tutor invites others to add to it: 'Gina has given us part of the answer here; who can add some more?'

Posing your own questions requires a little thought. It is important to configure a question that is comprehensible to the tutor – one to which others might also perhaps wish to hear an answer – and to ensure that this is a question, not a comment. Students frequently mix up the two, leaving the tutor unsure how best to respond, or at worst feeling that their teaching has been undermined. Here is Stewart (one of our case study nursing students) posing a very successful question associated with a lecture on cancer and altered body image:

> *I was interested in the points that you made about the sort of cancer which patients have and the effect of this on their body image. Some tumours are especially threatening. I've recently nursed a man who had a mouth cancer and he has had to have radical surgery. I wondered whether cancers that affect the face are always more distressing?*

In this example, Stewart does three things. First, he orientates the tutor to where his question is focused: 'I was interested in the points that you made about …'. Second, he gives the briefest rationale for posing the question: 'I've recently nursed a man …'. Then he poses the question itself: 'I wondered whether …'. Stewart may already have a good idea that patients with head and neck cancers suffer a higher incidence of altered body image – he has witnessed their distress. But he still manages to phrase this as a question that the tutor can answer and others can understand.

Activity 4.5   Reflection

In the next lecture that you attend, pay particular attention to the ways in which questions are posed by students. Does the quality of questioning significantly enhance what you take away from a lecture? What do you think that the student who asks questions takes away from the session that other students might not? Rather tellingly, Fatima observed to me once, 'A lecture is a performance, but it's not only that of the lecturer. Sometimes students perform too.'

As this answer is based on your own observation, there is no outline answer at the end of the chapter.

After the lecture has finished

Beyond the lecture, there remains other work to be done. Here is my 'to do' list:

- Expand on your notes in order to produce a resource that can assist you with assessments. You may need to consult a textbook to clarify your thinking at this point, or perhaps lecture notes that the teacher may have posted on the course web page. Writing points out as paragraphs forces you to express your reasoning in ways that real-time lecture notes cannot. Remember that in Chapter 3, I highlighted the value of speculation as part of higher-level critical thinking, so do not be afraid to include questions and possible ideas about what might be important, what might be happening in your notes.
- Identify any things that you do not understand. Where will you find fuller explanations? Perhaps this is something that will be available through a discussion in your tutor group. It is unwise to assume that a lecture will have explained everything and that you will be left query-free. Recognising what you do not yet know is part of that which drives future learning.
- Make a reflective note concerning your perceptions at this point. If you found some of the arguments made by the tutor unsettling or startling, determine why this is. What within your past experience, attitudes or values led you to alternative perspectives? What, if anything, needs to change now?

Chapter summary

Lectures are probably the learning opportunity that students think they know the most about and sometimes learn the least from. Overexposure to lectures, as well as making assumptions that one can get by frantically note-taking about everything, can undermine what can be achieved by full engagement with a lecture. Lectures are a common feature within nursing courses, so it is foolish not to derive the maximum benefit from them. By engaging with the lecture and its subject matter, you can learn a great deal and contribute to the successful learning of others. This chapter has highlighted how framing can serve to improve your engagement with what the lecturer offers. It has outlined how the questions that you then pose, as well as answer, materially enrich everyone's learning. Critically evaluating what the lecturer says exercises you in the sort of higher-level thinking that will be valued by assessors in your coursework later.

Preparing carefully for the lecture and following up with polished notes will significantly enhance what you learn. Materially, though, it is perhaps the quality of thinking within the lecture that determines whether you will develop the inquisitive attitudes that are so important in nursing. In the lecture, you witness the reasoning of another – the tutor.

Activities: brief outline answers

Activity 4.2   Reflection (page 71)

It's worth pausing to reflect on what happens as you learn from lectures. The process of learning involves re-examining knowledge, beliefs and attitudes as well as developing new ones. Whatever the lecturer imagines, it's unlikely that they can simply inculcate you in beliefs, values and attitudes that they commend. The lecture will at times create a dissonance for you, between what you believe now and what you might in the future. We all build slightly different templates for good practice. We cannot readily abandon values or beliefs that have been developed over time, that linked to culture, experience or past teaching.

What we must do, however, is ensure that our developing beliefs and values accord with the code of practice set down by the Nursing and Midwifery Council (2018a). In particular, we must respect the individuality and the dignity of patients. Imagine then that the lecturer has described a series of values about person-centred care and patients partnering the nurse in care planning. The lecturer believes that patients should engage fully in care planning. You believe that this is only possible some of the time. Some patients wish to be passive consumers of care. You are not required to blindly adopt the lecturer's values relating to person-centred care, but you cannot shirk the responsibility of what follows next. How much should the nurse press the patient to co-plan nursing care if some are reluctant to collaborate? At that point, meeting the NMC code requires you balance beliefs about what ideally happens (professional philosophy) with what could seem possible for the patient. This becomes a moment where theory and practice meet (a test of the utility of ideas) and it is a moment when values are reconsidered.

It's an excellent idea to consult on doubts and issues that emerge in a lecture, within a tutorial. Here there is greater scope to compare different perspectives and recommendations. In my experience, if you frame the forthcoming lecture well, with preparatory reading, you will then be in a better position at tutorial to explain what seemed controversial within the lecture and what seems commendable thereafter.

Activity 4.4   Critical thinking (page 74)

I think three things are important when it comes to note-taking in lectures. First, from the outset, you should learn to trust your own thinking. If the course is simply perceived as an exercise in collecting information, you are much more likely to write coursework assignments that are criticised for being too descriptive. Tutors want you to think. Your notes in the lecture, then, should consist of thoughts, with the briefest prompts from what the lecture has provided. The second important thing is to connect what you think to what was taught. This is why it is good to arrange the note page in three columns so that you can link a handout to what you wrote down. The third thing is to successfully connect this lecture to follow-up work, perhaps some reading or a tutorial discussion. This is why the third column on the notes page is so important.

I strongly recommend expanding your lecture notes after the session has finished. Writing out fuller sentences and paragraphs reinforces the learning from the session and makes revision much easier. A handout and brief notes will seem less clear several months later. If you work consistently in this way, building a note-taking approach and writing up points afterwards, you will develop an excellent reasoning and revision aid.

Further reading

Kirschner, P and Hendrick, C (2020) *How learning happens: seminal works in educational psychology and what they mean for practice*. Abingdon: Routledge.

There is a comparative dearth of accessible textbook help on the evolution of attitudes, values and beliefs through the process of learning. Most popular texts on the subject are self-help and designed to enhance motivation and build business success: little is written about what challenges arise in the areas we study. This book though is worth dipping into if you wish to understand more about the ways in which reasoning changes, including that related to attitudes and values. Chapter 6 discusses how new knowledge is shaped by existing knowledge and Chapter 10 reflects on achievement, that which we believe is merit worthy. This is a valuable book for tutors, and it has brief insights for curious students too.

McPherson, F (2020) *Effective notetaking*, 3rd edition. Wellington: Wayz Press.

Fiona McPherson offers a comprehensive review of different note-taking strategies, including the use of concept analysis and spider diagrams. The argument runs that if you transform your notes into a different and perhaps more visual form, you reinforce learning and build connections to other subject matters. This is a useful book for students and tutors alike, and could also help to shape lecture designs.

Useful websites

https://youtu.be/hl-2TxkEwn0

How to take effective lecture notes-my best note-taking tips and tools. Prep with Jen.

In this short video, Jen offers you an alternative way to set out your lecture notes and useful ideas on how to signpost what within them you need to return to when writing up the material more fully. There is a greater emphasis here on rehearsing information so that can be replicated later. While that remains true within nursing (for instance remembering the circulation of the heart) your learning will often have to seem more quizzical. I would encourage you then to add notes debating claims made within a lecture and what that might mean for practice.

www.youtube.com/watch?v=Y9LBUf1NzU0

How to improve your listening skills.

As the speaker in this video on how to improve your listening skills suggests, we all think we know how to listen effectively, but he makes a persuasive case that this is not always the case. It is well worth reviewing the video to improve your chances of securing the most from the nursing lectures that you attend. Do not worry that the examples do not come from nursing – the principles still apply.

Chapter 5 Making sense of interactive enquiries

Chapter aims

After reading this chapter, you will be able to:

- describe the key features of interactive enquiry;
- indicate how you need to prepare for and attend to the different learning opportunities offered there;
- contrast learning in these settings with that in the lecture.

Introduction

Every nursing course has a structure, a mix of learning activities that contribute to the whole. Lecturing provides a substantial amount of the teaching in most courses.

Other smaller group-based and more interactive enquiries are also part of your course, encouraging learning by doing, discussing or speculating (Wong, 2018). Terminology may vary from course to course, but I suggest that you may encounter variants of the following:

- Module tutorials: led by the module tutor or their associates and typically in a small group setting. The tutorials may do different things, but typically this includes reviewing lecture series and their fit to the module's intended learning outcomes, to practise placements and to forthcoming assessments. It is through module tutorials that you should sense the design of the course. Personal tutorials are different and may be run one to one or else in a small group of perhaps three to four students. Personal tutors work to help you master study skills across the course (Grey and Osborne, 2020).
- Seminars: Seminars typically link reading from the library and your module studies. Seminars might also focus upon enquiries in clinical practice (Jakobsen and Maehre, 2023). For example, within a seminar you might each present case studies of care and discuss what they reveal. In seminars you discover information and present it to colleagues, learning from each other as well as a supervising tutor.
- Workshops imply more collaborative learning and they typically include some element of trying out ideas and discovery. An expert might demonstrate a skill (a masterclass, Mitrea et al., 2022), but just as frequently you might find solutions of your own working as a group. Workshops can focus upon interpersonal skills in which case role play may make an important contribution. For example, you might have a role-play workshop on responding to anxious or aggressive patients.
- Skills laboratory sessions. You will need to learn a range of psychomotor skills (ways to use your hands, to practise safely and deftly) and these are typically arranged in a skills laboratory or explored through computer-based simulation programmes (Nakayoshi et al., 2021). While they include skilled demonstrations of procedures (such as cleaning a tracheostomy) there is still an element of trying procedures out so that you appreciate what is required to practise sensitively.

Activity 5.1 Reflection

Look back now to Table 3.1 and 3.2 in Chapter 3 (pages 49–51) and determine how many of the ascending skills detailed there depend strongly upon the above forms of interactive study.

Because this is a personal reflection activity, no suggested answer is offered at the end of the chapter.

My guess is that interactive learning will seem vital to your progress. In my experience such studies incur greater anxiety for students, but they promise greater rewards if you can overcome worries about contributing. One of the key challenges you might face is trusting the idea that you can learn from and with fellow students. The second key challenge concerns overcoming the feeling that if 'they simply taught me this' it would be so much faster. Interactive studies are set precisely because tutors hope to help you reason more flexibly and proactively (Koivisto et al., 2016; K.-C. Lee et al., 2018). Nursing practice will demand such reasoning of you repeatedly.

Interactive enquiries serve a very important role as you work towards forming the templates for nursing care. They help you to develop the ability to make a case of your own and conduct debates (Gambrill and Gibbs, 2017). These forms of learning activity permit no hiding place from the responsibility to decide some things for yourself. In clinical practice, care is negotiated and consulted upon. You will have to express professional values and argue for what seems to be the best care.

So, what characterises interactive enquiries?

- You are often set tasks and given limited briefs. The study requires enquiry, within the library and beyond.
- You will need to liaise with your fellow students. A tutor or librarian will guide you, but they will not tell you what to think.
- You will need to structure your enquiries, the information gathering, sifting and sorting, and that which is discovered.
- You will need to communicate in a collegiate way.

Gina had the following to say about this sort of learning activity:

I found the interactive group learning difficult at first. I think that was down to two things. First, it seemed to require so much more effort. Tutors were acquainting us with the insecurity of practice reasoning in as safe a way as they could. The second reason it seemed tough was that the group work required me to trust other students. It could feel as though the blind were leading the blind. The best tutors though knew when to step in and signal that we were off down a pointless path.

Activity 5.2   Reflection

Make a list now of the expectations that you think you should fairly have of fellow students engaged in interactive studies with you. In your experience are these usually met? Next list what tutors do to help the studies seem constructive.

My suggestions appear at the end of the chapter.

Learning from role play

Fatima told me that she hates role-play learning. She was quite emphatic about the matter: 'If I wanted to act, I would have gone to drama school!' Her anxiety is entirely normal. When role playing, you risk discovering things about how you think at exactly the time as they are exhibited to the others involved. By role play, I mean a carefully orchestrated and time-limited interaction of a group of students (and sometimes others), each of whom has a defined role to play while exploring a process, circumstance, opportunity or problem that is relevant in nursing. The role play includes a briefing, a period of interaction where you enter the role and imagine how care might seem, and then afterwards a period of debrief where you take stock of the experience (Presti, 2019). To make role play feel more accessible, it is important to acknowledge that you are trying out ideas, interactions, ways to express care. Role play might help you to uncover some deeply held attitudes, values and beliefs. Aydin Er et al. (2017) detail just how important nursing values are to students in nursing. Your tutor will encourage fellow students to reflect on the episode with you, about your role, in a constructive and encouraging way.

In role play, the tutor remains attentive, ready to call a timeout so that you can share a conversation about any issues that arise. Sometimes you may be asked to be the observer of a colleague's role play, providing them with thoughtful feedback. A skilful tutor will allow the role play to develop for several minutes and will then help you to pick out some observations about what was happening. Key points might attend to:

- whether the activity was proceeding as anticipated (why or why not?);
- whether you felt comfortable with what you were doing or saying;
- whether you felt that you understood what another person did or said;
- whether there are other ways in which you could have handled a particular interaction.

Table 5.1 details some critical thinking benefits of role-play learning that I think you should consider.

I asked Fatima and Raymet what they found helped them to prepare for role play. Below is what they told me – I have also annotated each response with reflections of my own.

Fatima

I need quite a lot of reassurance about role play, especially if there is a new tutor leading the session. For that reason, I make a point of checking with the tutor beforehand what the purpose of the role play is.

It is important that the tutor sets out the purpose and the planned process for role-play learning sessions. I sometimes say to students that they are not yet qualified nurses, so this is a form of play, much as happens in childhood. Here, we can try out ideas, and perspectives. Even if they must later be modified to be acceptable, we can do that in a very supportive way. The role play is a learning activity, not an assessment. You cannot fail it, but you might need to do some extra thinking based on insights gained. You are allowed to signal when explorations seem too much, or you need a break.

Role-play feature	Critical thinking benefit
Imagining yourself in the role of another (e.g. a distressed relative)	We rarely rehearse the experiences, perceptions and approaches of others. In role play, you see how emotional contexts help to shape interactions, something that you have read about as a higher-order feature of reasoning in Chapter 1.
Focusing upon professionally relevant interactions	It is very difficult for theory to seem practice-authentic. Learning on campus seems to operate in a privileged place. Role play focuses on relatively discrete interactions that enable us to anticipate how care in action might seem. Seeing what is realistically possible teaches us about what nurses focus upon, how they negotiate care.
Exploring beliefs and values, those you imagine others might use	Beliefs and values shape a great deal in healthcare, although they are not necessarily analysed in everyday clinical conversations. Role playing situations of tension or conflict can help us to analyse how we and others approach the world around us. Because we acted 'in role' with support, we can then review the insights gained.
Exercising safe decisions about what to do next	In Part 1, I emphasised the importance of developing templates, ways in which nurses enact care, weighing up what is realistic. It would seem daunting to have to do that again and again in practice from scratch. In role play, we can try out solutions and examine what seemed to work best.
Reacting in real time to how others behave	In Chapter 2, we briefly explored why reflection in action is more difficult. Hindsight helps us to improve upon our reasoning. Role play, with its debrief, provides both forms of reflective activity.
Comparing experience with research/teaching/theory	Nursing information, ideas and plans need to be realistic. In role play, you have the chance to try out what it takes to express a theory, to use teaching or research findings.
Exploring the emotional labour of practice	Nursing work can seem draining as we have to demonstrate emotional intelligence, working with the needs and perspectives of others. Understanding what may seem most tiring is important if you are to think and act strategically.

Table 5.1 Features of role play and critical thinking benefits

Raymet

I've found that how well I do in role-play sessions depends on how stressed I am before the session, whether I perhaps feel tense about something else entirely. Then I say to myself, 'This is pretend time.' The easiest role plays for me are where the roles, the situations, are entirely new to me. Then I don't have baggage to expose, at least any that I'm aware of.

Notice Raymet's concern about role play as a performance – she wants to act well. Role play, though, is simply a vehicle for learning and it will require some focused imaginative work. You need to be sincere in imagining what the role entails. Raymet makes an excellent point about fresh situations. If we role play there, our 'performance' might be less polished, but there seems to be less risk that we will reveal something which we have doubts about. My recommendation is to write up reflections on the role play, including your feelings and insights, after the session has ended.

Activity 5.3   Critical thinking

Jot down now some practice situations that you think it would be good to explore in class using role play.

Discuss these with your fellow students to see if you have common needs. Consider asking your module tutor to see if selected role plays could then be arranged.

As this answer is based on your own observation, there is no outline answer at the end of the chapter.

Learning within seminars

Interaction is also equally important in seminars, another form of group learning. In a seminar, individual students are briefed to fulfil different information-gathering tasks within the literature or on the internet, and to bring back their discoveries to the group (Morgan, 2019; Strawson et al., 2021). Seminars are typically small group activities so that all can participate.

Seminars are designed to teach you study skills (especially those relating to search and find), project management skills (you need to work to a common project end) and critical thinking skills (a weighing up of evidence and options available). You will need to be disciplined in your work and brave enough to report your discoveries. Because everyone is asked to contribute in this way, seminars also teach you that you can learn from fellow students as well as your tutor.

Activity 5.4   Group work

As it takes a little while to build confidence as a seminar learner, you might find it useful to practise this work informally with some of your fellow students before you tackle a bigger exercise within a class. Choose a health-related news story reported in the press. Next, each take a different newspaper that reports the story and summarise what is focused upon, how the issue is portrayed. Then report your findings back to an informal student group to gain an understanding of how stories may vary. Did all of the newspapers identify the same issues? This is what a seminar involves – the gathering and critical comparison of information.

As this answer is based on your own observation, there is no outline answer at the end of the chapter.

During the search stage of any seminar work, you will need to find the best possible literature or website information to share. If you bring back something that is not quite clear, more discussion work will be needed at the end. During the report and discussion stage of the seminar, it is important to present a clear summary of your discovery and what you make of it. Afterwards, you will need to stand ready with constructive questions for those who present their work (e.g. 'How confident do you feel about the author's claims?').

Seminar work challenges you to: discriminate (e.g. about what material to use); interpret (e.g. about what authors really argue); speculate (e.g. regarding what might be the significance of evidence uncovered); and make arguments (e.g. regarding what care now seems justified). Your tutor is likely to work within the seminar group to help you do a number of things:

- determine that what you seem to be concluding, or what you agree for the time being, remains uncertain (summarising);
- explore other questions and consider alternative perspectives;
- identify when your discussions are going 'off-track' – the tutor's contributions, though, will often remain speculative in nature and they will be at pains not to instruct you.

Stewart and I discussed his approach to preparing for seminar work. It may give you confidence to learn that Stewart consistently achieved A or B grades in his coursework, with tutors highlighting his ability to successfully organise information. I have listed his commendable suggestions:

1. Do not prevaricate – searching for information takes more time than you might imagine. Don't be afraid to ask the librarian for help.

2. Ask the tutor to clarify the focus of the seminar before you proceed to search for information. Some of the best seminars are arranged in terms of answers to a set question.

3. Collaborate quickly and regularly. Sometimes you will work alone to bring information back to a seminar, but quite often the search work is shared. If so, check that you have the means to contact one another – that way you can minimise the risk that information is missed or duplicated.

4. Make meticulous notes as regards the source material. It is frustrating to try to locate work with inadequate references later.

5. Jot down your questions as you read. Do this immediately after you have read a piece of literature.

6. Do not be afraid to acknowledge gaps in your knowledge after your search work is completed. Other students may bring back information that fills in a gap for you. In any case, some areas of healthcare have a patchy evidence base.

Learning within workshops

Workshops are often designed to facilitate problem solving and then they usually start with patient care scenarios (Compton et al., 2020). You and your colleagues are invited to use available evidence to work out what the important issues are, what is problematic, and how you will then proceed (e.g. managing a patient's chronic pain).

What typically distinguishes a workshop from a seminar is that it centres on how to combine different elements of information, wedding research evidence, experience and skills review together, for example. While the seminar classically emphasises reading within the literature, a workshop might ask you to interview practitioners on their care strategies, perhaps requiring you to review healthcare policies and link them to recent research. A workshop often operates more closely to the sort of template thinking that you first read about in Chapter 1. Raymet came to like workshop learning. She noted:

Nursing is untidy, work never complete, and workshop learning assures me that others see it that way too. It was a relief to understand you don't necessarily solve problems alone.

Activity 5.5   Reflection

Here are two areas where I have helped students within a workshop approach. Each required the marrying of information, skills and practice context insights. On each occasion, I introduced one or more clinicians to enhance the learning opportunities for students. Why do you think each was especially suited to a workshop approach?

1. Helping patients to come to terms with having a permanent colostomy after surgery for bowel cancer.
2. Helping patients to make sense of their anxiety disorder.

An outline answer is given at the end of this chapter.

Raymet and I agree that workshop learning works best when three things happen. First, there is a sense of achievement linked to the discoveries made, both personal and those that the group managed between them. So, begin by expecting to discover something personally important that you can share. Second, there is surprise at what is discovered through group work (about the subject but also collective endeavour). Third, there is pleasure in working with others within a group that seems to 'gel'. Nursing emphasises teamwork and collaboration, as well as learning from experience, so workshops are an important way of learning. The ability to develop and then demonstrate independent thought, right at the top of the critical thinking and reflective reasoning hierarchy, is closely associated with a willingness to collaborate towards shared discoveries.

Managing uncertainty

At the heart of all interactive enquiry is the need to manage uncertainty. What is required of us, of me, and what shall we do to manage the project set before us? What might be achieved, missed or perhaps misunderstood? What mistakes might happen to confuse our understanding of a subject? If we can manage uncertainty, learning becomes more pleasurable.

If interactive enquiry left no uncertainty, no issues to debate, there would be no scope for learning through experience. We would not understand what effort it takes to reach decisions or to make policies or protocols, and we would not understand how groups can operate together to develop strategies of their own. Fatima felt the uncertainty of her interactive enquiry learning activities acutely. She observed:

> *What alarmed me was not only just how much we didn't know, but how unsettling it was then to agree on the best ways to act. I craved assurance and only gradually learned to trust our group to make good decisions.*

Activity 5.6   Critical thinking

Look at the following list of possible ways of resolving interactive learning uncertainty and decide which of these could have helped you with past problems. That experience may come from a past course or even outside of nursing – the principles still hold good.

- Ask the tutor/group adviser to clarify the project brief before you set off.
- Check what arrangements are in place for ensuring that work proceeds in the right direction.
- Set out a schedule of work, agreeing what sorts of activities are needed and who will be responsible for each.
- Agree a means of recording your progress, the decisions agreed, and the discoveries made.
- Determine group etiquette (i.e. an agreed way of talking about each other's contributions).

As this answer is based on your own observation, there is no outline answer at the end of the chapter.

To complete your interactive enquiry activities, it is necessary to start with the clearest possible brief (Strawson et al., 2021). If yours seems unclear, you should ask your tutor to clarify points for you. In most instances, group activities are supported by a written brief. Within a problem-based learning exercise, for example, there is likely to be one or more patient case studies and associated tasks to complete (Compton et al., 2020). Typically, too, the project will set out the aims and objectives of the exercise so that you can sense what work is necessary.

While tutors do not direct the work of the group, they are required to monitor your work. Consulting with the tutor on a regular basis in projects that span several weeks is important.

Project groups are usually composed of people with a mix of aptitudes, and it is certainly not expected that all group members will be good at everything. To benefit, however, you will need to be prepared to volunteer what you feel comfortable doing, even if you believe your work might not be perfect. You will also need to acknowledge the work done by others who have other talents. Setting aside personal insecurities is part of the learning process. Start with the assumption that we all have insecurities, many of which are unspoken. What is more important now is that what you share works to achieve project ends.

Wasted time increases the pressures on a group, especially as they near the point where they must present their findings. For that reason, agreeing a schedule of work, as well as how much time is allocated to each part of the project, helps to discipline the enquiry. Instead of a project that finishes with a lot of information about just one thing, you will have a project that seems balanced and measured. It is then necessary to keep a brief record of the lines of enquiry and the decisions made. Such an 'audit trail' enables the group to tell the story of their enquiry, as well as presenting the end product of what they have learned.

Chapter summary

Interactive enquiry activities represent some of the most active learning that you are likely to engage in. Interactive learning is proactive, challenging you to engage with project tasks, contributing questions and solutions as you proceed. While they require significant personal effort and imagination, they have the benefit of bridging the gap between theory and practice. Role play, for example, simulates the untidiness of clinical conversation. If you elect to conduct role plays on concerns that have arisen while on clinical placements, you will find that they quickly become engaging.

Seminars and workshops emphasise learning within the group. You will learn as much about the process and enquiry as about the subject matter of the project work shared. You will need to be well organised here, diligent, and consultative. Reasoning in these contexts requires more collaboration and effort. It is an investment well made, however. Much of the nursing you will practise later relies upon just such shared learning.

Activities: brief outline answers

Activity 5.2   Reflection (page 81)

I would expect other students to:

*   Approach enquiries seriously and diligently. If they don't then additional work falls on others and the reputation of the group suffers.
*   Respect different reports and opinions shared within the group (it is yet to be established what seems the wisest interpretation of information).

- Show patience and consideration to others who struggle with some element of the project. We are all likely to discover weaknesses as well as strengths through study.
- Use questions to interrogate information rather than people. The goal is to examine what information can teach us and what remains to be understood.
- Respect collective decisions within the group, for example about when to consult a tutor.

Unfortunately, not all students feel equally committed to interactive enquiry. This might be a serious matter because if a colleague is unwilling to collaborate now, will they find it any easier to consult well in clinical practice? As a last resort it may be necessary to complain to tutorial staff about a colleague who disrupts or undermines group learning. Tutors are adept at reading group communication and body language messages, so don't be surprised if periodically they call 'time out' and revisit with you any group etiquette rules set down. While students have different learning styles and preferences it would be unwise to imagine that interactive learning can be simply discarded. Much of the fabric of successful nursing practice relies on collaboration and teamwork.

Activity 5.5   Reflection (page 86)

Helping patients to come to terms with having a permanent colostomy after surgery for bowel cancer

The workshop approach was especially useful in this instance because my clinical colleague offered brief illustrations of how she talked about stomas to patients, and I added some theory on changes to body image caused by bowel cancer. We then invited the students to review questions that patients had asked about their colostomy and discussed the best ways to answer these.

Helping patients to make sense of their anxiety disorder

In this workshop, the students first generated ideas about admission to hospital that they believed would worry patients with a pre-existing anxiety disorder. A clinical psychologist then explored with the students how they had selected their ideas and why they believed hospital admission might cause alarm. I acted as secretary to the group, recording the conclusions reached, and then related that to the theory of risk assessment.

Further reading

Heinrich, P (2018) *When role play comes alive: a theory and practice.* London: Palgrave Macmillan.

Paul Heinrich is an unashamed advocate of role play in healthcare, and I share that enthusiasm. There is considerable scope to use role play to enhance the compassion base of nurse education.

Useful websites

https://youtu.be/SArAggTULLU

Fox, P Adult learning theory: Knowles' 6 assumptions of adult learners.

I want to encourage you to use this video clip to examine some of the assumptions (from Knowles) that are likely to underpin many of the interactive enquiries that you engage in upon your course. If you are a student, reference to these assumptions should help you provide better feedback to tutors. Are activities, for instance, well structured so that the purpose of study is clear? As a student, it's important to ask, how well do I match Knowles' assumptions about adult learning? Do I need a degree of freedom to enquire, to follow leads that intrigue me?

Do I secure a sense of achievement through collaborative enquiry? If you are struggling with interactive studies these six assumptions might be a good thing to discuss with your personal tutor. While nurses learn individually they also need to work collectively as well. Educational psychology is obviously of interest to your tutor, but it is relevant to you as well, as you differentiate learning challenges and opportunities.

Chapter 6   Making clinical placements successful

NMC Future Nurse: Standards of Proficiency for Registered Nurses

This chapter will address the following platforms and proficiencies:

Platform 1: Being an accountable professional

At the point of registration, the registered nurse will be able to:

1.8   Demonstrate the knowledge, skills and ability to think critically when applying evidence and drawing on experience to make evidence informed decisions in all situations.

1.18   Demonstrate the knowledge and confidence to contribute effectively and pro-actively in an interdisciplinary team.

Platform 3: Assessing needs and planning care

At the point of registration, the registered nurse will be able to:

3.15   Demonstrate the ability to work in partnership with people, families and carers to continuously monitor, evaluate and reassess the effectiveness of all agreed nursing care plans and care, sharing decision making and readjusting agreed goals, documenting progress and decisions made.

Chapter aims

After reading this chapter, you will be able to:

- summarise the nature of critical enquiry that you need to engage in within clinical placements;
- detail what preparations will enable you to complete a successful clinical placement;
- discuss the part played by the student–practice supervisor relationship in a satisfying and effective learning placement;
- understand the reflective and open approach you must use if feedback is to aid your studies.

Introduction

Recently I shared a conversation with Sue, our case study registered nurse, and Phillip, a junior doctor, about what was required to learn within a new clinical placement. Here are the things that they told me about, which may 'ring true' for you as well:

- Learning always involves a degree of difficult adjustment but students develop a patterned way of coping. First, you learn the routines of the workplace, the etiquette and the protocols that operate there. Hagg-Martinell et al. (2016) characterise this as learning about the 'community of practice'. This is akin to creating a map, helping you to understand what might happen on a typical shift.
- After this has been established you then embark upon learning the additional contextual information, that related to the clinical specialism, its group of patients and their needs.
- Alongside that and stretching beyond, learners start to understand the ways in which clinicians manage the many different demands upon them, providing safe and equitable care. The way this is done is to profile the recurring patient needs and the ways that clinicians anticipated these. To that is added information about treatments and risk management. In Chapter 1 of this book, I called these templates.

Activity 6.1   Evaluation

Look back now to what you learned in Chapter 2 about the simple reflective practice model that asked, 'what', 'so what' and what next?' (pp 29, Rolfe et al., 2011). Does this set of questions illuminate what Sue and Phillip suggest as an order of learning work in practice?

I offer my brief thoughts at the end of the chapter.

Later, Sue explained that learners had to also manage the obvious gap between theory and practice (Hediye and Seher, 2022). Some of what was celebrated on campus didn't seem possible in practice. Much of what was done in practice didn't receive considerate attention on campus (e.g. equitably managing care budgets and time allocation). Students then might adopt one of three explanatory narratives.

- The first was that practice was ill equipped to meet the standards commended on campus (resource deficit narrative).
- The second narrative (and logical opposite) was that theory was hopelessly naïve and pursued ideals that were impracticable (the idealism deficit narrative).
- The third, and the one that Sue commended, was the utility narrative (Dolan et al., 2022). This put theory at the service of the practitioner and acknowledged that difficult decisions would always have to be made. If, though, you abandoned theory,

then you got stuck within custom and that was lazy or even dangerous. Theory fuelled imagination and that too was important if practice was to change.

I argue that practice placements are a key resource as you learn templates that are ethical, evidence related, person centred and practicable. Practice placements acquaint you with notions of service as well as examples of care (e.g. De Bruin et al., 2021). If you are to discover such templates though, you will need to engage in some pattern recognition. Don't worry – you are already very good at it. Your brain has developed to notice what seems to fit with what (Smith et al., 2015). Human beings are predisposed to look for order in chaos. However, because clinical environments offer a significant volume of stimuli, experiences that you can attend to, there is merit in asking you to work in a slightly more methodical way. Instead of trying to practise all the reasoning attributes you read about in Chapter 1 at once, it is useful to begin with Rolfe et al. (2011) recommended questions (see Table 6.1).

What?	Imagine that your placement is in a health clinic and its work is with a range of people dealing with chronic illnesses. The focus of work centres upon rehabilitation but also thereafter health maintenance. Staff hope to help patients retain independence. Staff are repeatedly engaged in demonstrations of techniques, teaching and counselling of patients. The priority need is to sustain patient trust, confidence and relevant self-care skills. Doing this reduces the need for emergency treatment and care later.
What seems the important work of this practice area, what does it centre upon? What is repeatedly done, according to protocol or norms? What remain the priority expressed needs related to this setting?	
So what?	This spotlights mutual care planning with patients and measures designed to motivate or teach them. While the chronic illnesses may vary the recurring work remains centred on the psychology of patient coping and the clinicians work in sustaining patient efforts to self-care. Nurses must be effective listeners and collaborative problem solvers. Liaison with family members is important too. Nurses must be able to explain the best research evidence available, that which sustains patient independence.
Once we understand the nature of work in the clinical setting, we focus upon what nurses actually do to answer demands arising there.	
What next?	Nurses engage in a variety of problem identification and resolution measures, and they carefully record the success or otherwise of collaboration with patients over time. The care relationship is seen in terms of years with periodic times of more intensive guidance offered. While there are commended ways to facilitate coping among patients, the staff are eager to audit trail past success or failure, insisting that patient profiles and needs cannot be entirely linked to standard treatment protocols. What works best depends both upon treatment innovation and upon patients' ability or motivation to adopt new self-care measures. Care becomes dynamic, investigative, and consultative in nature.
The focus on nursing work moves towards skills that make care work successful. The combination of knowledge and skills become working templates.	

Table 6.1   Reflective Practice questions to help open clinical learning (after Rolfe et al., 2011; MTa Learning, 2021)

> ## Activity 6.2   Reflection
>
> Study Table 6.1 now to determine whether you think the three reflective questions help you focus on:
>
> a)   what the nurses are doing in the health clinic example offered, and;
>
> b)   what practice templates might look like.
>
> Your placement objectives will include some module-related requirements, and perhaps work to improve particular skills, but why might the focus upon understanding practice templates help bring understanding together?
>
> *I offer brief points for your consideration at the end of the chapter.*

Building a clinical case study

Nursing care is not delivered through fragmented care episodes; it is arranged as part of the care relationship. If all we do is complete technical procedures that are necessary for treatment, then much is lost. To understand this fully, there is merit in studying an individual patient's changing needs, during the course of your placement, or a significant part thereof. Historically, such profile studies of patients and their needs led to the writing up of 'nursing care studies'. Today, case studies are being written for new purposes, such as to better explore an unusual patient problem (Cadet, 2018), a nursing skill in action, or what it means to deliver person-centred care (Price, 2022).

If you negotiate to study a case study patient's care during the placement the following are important:

- Case study learning must be sanctioned by your practice supervisor and fit with the requirements of your module of study. The purpose of the case study is to illuminate patient-distinctive needs and the ways in these are addressed. A case study can illustrate where, how, when and why care departs from what is offered as routine.
- You must ask the patient's permission to focus enquiries on their care. You are not acting as a researcher, but rather as a reflective practitioner. You will need to ask the patient more about their experiences, what they expect of care, and how they try to liaise with the nurses and doctors. It is necessary to acquaint them with any particular focus of interest that you have. For example, perhaps the patient is coming to terms with a chronic illness, so you are especially interested in how they learn about the illness and useful self-care measures.
- The partner patient should be someone who feels comfortable discussing their circumstances and work with care staff to address their needs. The ideal patient is probably inquisitive about their care, and they feel able to articulate their experiences.

- The patient needs to remain in your care sufficiently long to better explore needs and care negotiation.
- The patient should be someone that your practice supervisor also cares for. While you deliver a percentage of their care, it is important that you are also able to access how the patient and the registered nurse interact.

Your clinical placement thereafter involves regular discussions with the patient and your practice supervisor to better understand how care evolves, as well as how needs are identified and addressed. In particular, it helps you to understand how each explains (narrates) the care in progress. Do they use the same language, for instance?

Your case-study note-taking will incrementally accumulate during the course of your placement. It should include:

- Questions and reflections about what you witness. Some of the notes will constitute full reflective practice episodes, but do not be afraid to jot down passing impressions as well.
- Queries about clinical reasoning, that which your practice supervisor might explain about problem solving.
- Summary of any related reading linked with your chosen case study.
- Periodic summaries of what you think you have discovered, which might (for example) entail detailing the order of teaching offered to a patient with a chronic illness, reviewing what the patient mastered quickly or struggled to understand, and exploring what the patient wanted to know compared with what seemed clinically necessary to teach.

Preparing for the placement

Preparation for your placement can significantly reduce anxieties, such as those about a busy work environment and the risk of making errors there (Rosina et al., 2022). The more you can bring order to the learning experience, working with your practice supervisor, the more constructive the learning will seem. Table 6.2 suggests what might be done in advance of your placement.

Strategy	Benefit
Review the learning outcomes that must be achieved during this placement and any assessment arrangements that apply. If you think studying a case study might assist you, alert your practice supervisor to that as part of your introduction.	You focus on what must be achieved. Practice supervisors want to show you a lot, but it can seem rather random. If you can help them to link enquiries to the discovery of important care templates, you may create a focus that excites both of you.
Research the work of the department, ward or practice by looking at any details on healthcare agency websites.	By doing some homework, you will not have to ask quite so many 'what?' questions on your placement.

(Continued)

Table 6.2   (Continued)

Strategy	Benefit
Revisit your portfolio to identify particular practice skills that you wish to improve on (e.g. patient history taking).	You calmly determine what needs your attention. Practice skills are important, they are the means through which, care is actioned, and templates realised.
Make personal contact with the clinical team, writing to or e-mailing the nurse in charge.	You establish an immediate rapport if you show such personal organisation.
Try to establish in advance who your practice supervisor will be.	Knowing this will increase your confidence.
Ascertain what sorts of illness, injury or other health challenges tax patients in the placement area.	The patients on a ward often share some common concerns and needs. This might assist you to identify possible clinical case study opportunities.
Check when your first shift is and arrive in good time, correctly attired.	

Table 6.2   Getting ready for clinical placement study

Working with your practice supervisor

Students are not always aware of what a supervisor brings to student support, so let us summarise that. Practice supervisors are experienced practitioners who are familiar with their area of care and its local policies and protocols. They have undertaken a short course in the principles of learning, teaching, support and assessment, and they are charged with guiding you during your clinical placement. They act as advocates of learning, but they also have responsibilities to inculcate you into the team and its work (Rosina et al., 2022). They work to help you master skills and apply your knowledge, but retain responsibilities towards their patients, colleagues and the profession. Practice supervisors share unique insights into the practical ways of conducting nursing work (Ryan and McAllister, 2020).

Successful work with your practice supervisor will:

- help you to manage your anxieties about learning in the clinical setting;
- help you to develop an acceptable approach to enquiry in this setting;
- open doors to other expertise in the clinical setting;
- give you thoughtful and honest weekly feedback so that you are well prepared for assessments and end-of-placement reports;
- help you to address your own learning agenda, as well as that required by the course.

The working relationship with your practice supervisor should be one of trust and mutual respect. Practice supervisors expect students to arrive ready and eager to learn. Judging how much learning to take on, as well as how fast, in a clinical context will need to be negotiated. It will be necessary to be honest with your practice supervisor as regards what you feel you can cope with. Some learning within placement will be opportunistic. If you engage in that learning, though, request a review discussion afterwards so that you can evaluate that which was witnessed. Other learning will be skills focused, and your practice supervisor will quite probably demonstrate several procedures – do not be afraid to ask about those afterwards.

Other learning opportunities within the clinical area may be carefully planned. Sue, for instance, describes how she briefs her students on those:

> *I have eight or nine recurring learning opportunities that I want all students to consider while they are on the ward, and I've explained my thinking about that to the other clinicians. For example, we have an office round, reviewing patients and their treatment, before we go and talk to them at their bedsides. I want the learner to listen to what is discussed but also to consider why we proceed in that way.*

Sometimes the insights gained acquaint you with difficult decisions relating to care priorities and resource allocation. Care has an etiquette dimension, one that enables professionals to work together. Your practice supervisor should take the opportunity to debrief you on these afterwards. In the above example, Sue explains that many students ask about practice as a 'managed performance'. The discussions with the patients at their bedsides are influenced by what is discussed in the office beforehand.

Working with a practice supervisor then is not just about the best enquiry, and template understanding. It is not simply about skill demonstrations either. A skilful practice supervisor will help you to understand the ways in which the team communicate and how service is conceived (Rosina et al., 2022). At times, this may raise ethical or logistical issues that seem startling, and these also deserve discussion with the practice supervisor. Sue observed:

> *When I first started looking after students, I worried that care had to look perfect. I believed that it had to be textbook fashion. Of course, that was impossible. Care episodes are shaped by patient requests and behaviour, as well as the resources available. At the end of a shift, all concerned, patients and clinicians decide what was achieved.*

Activity 6.3 Reflection

Think back to a practice supervisor that you have admired and decide how important the following were to their success in that role. Do you identify any recurring support needs that you could alert future practice supervisors to?

- Creating a structure for the placement, key study opportunities or people to work with.
- Being ready to rehearse aloud how they reason care.
- Seeming empathetic, recalling learning anxieties and needs of their own.
- Offering a little challenge, prompting you to reason yourself before offering answers.
- Teaching you local etiquette and protocols so that you can quickly learn with the clinical team.

Because this is a personal reflection for you, no answer has been added at the chapter end.

Managing assessment

At the end of your placement, a practice assessor (one of the staff) will write up a report on your learning there. Reports cover matters such as the development of your skills, the attitudes that you demonstrate in practice, your commitment to nursing care and the gains made in your knowledge (Feeney and Everett, 2020). Today, assessment is said to be 'continuous', and we need to consider the psychology of this process, which can seem daunting.

There does need to be judgement on performance, and this remains an issue for qualified nurses. Annual staff appraisals, complaints by patients, and reviews by auditors are all part of professional life (NMC, 2019). Assessments that are made of your performance are mediated by an understanding of your stage of training and the learning objectives set. Importantly, good assessment takes account of your readiness to critically examine your own work. Insight is important, as well as practice performance (Walsh and Dixon, 2021). The staff are interested in your learning and your response to guidance. While you might demonstrate shortfalls in skill or knowledge, these can sometimes be compensated for by a willingness to receive instruction.

To help you manage assessment, you need to be critical of your own performance. You will need to recognise misconceptions that are not serving you well. Such a personal audit of week-by-week performance will then enable you to seek the guidance of your supervisor, and at the earliest possible point to start correcting any shortfalls and building on your successes. The following represent a series of week-by-week questions that might help you to evaluate your progress:

- What do you think was the best of my work this week and what still needed improvement?
- If you were to suggest one focus for improving my practice next week, what would it be and why?
- How do you think it feels for a patient to be nursed by me?

Assessments of your performance during a clinical placement will focus on your skills, the way in which you apply your knowledge, and your attitudes and values (Walsh and Dixon, 2021). The judgement of skills is usually well received by student nurses. Students understand that the practice supervisor and others who contribute to the assessment of your performance are skilful. Receiving critique of your applied knowledge is also usually well received, at least where the supervisor and others have asked you pertinent questions. It seems fair to critique applied knowledge where you have had the opportunity to reason aloud and demonstrate why you proceed as you do. Assessment of attitudes and values, however, can be contentious, and it sometimes feels hurtful. This is because your attitudes and values are inferred from what you do, what you say, and how you approach care and colleague relationships. When students struggle in this area of their learning, skilful coaching may need to follow.

Pause to reflect on how different the campus and the clinical environment are as places of learning. The robust enquiry and debate attitude that is so important on campus might seem aggressive in practice. Absolute thinking, something that we equated in Chapter 3 with lower levels of critical thinking and reflection, may in practice become a stereotype applied to patients or professional colleagues. It is vital that nurses learn to explore and respect the concerns of others. Remember that transitional thinking is characterised by the consideration of different possibilities. This, at the absolute minimum, is what you should be aiming for.

One of the ways to demonstrate your positive attitudes and values relating to care is to seize opportunities to discuss care philosophy with your supervisor and other senior staff. If you demonstrate an enquiring and respectful interest in what is being done, you are much more likely to convey favourable impressions to others. Students are usually well evaluated where both compassion and humility are demonstrated. To evaluate others as 'wrong', 'stupid' or 'naive' is likely to convey an arrogant attitude.

Whatever you claim regarding your attitudes and values, though, remember that deeds speak louder than words. Have you worn your uniform correctly? Have you been punctual? Have you shown a due degree of flexibility as regards what others need to do? Are you polite? How do others know that you are listening attentively to what they tell you? The patterns of shifts that you complete as a student on placement are a foretaste of what work will feel like. For nurses to trust you as a colleague, they must feel sure that you will attend on time and work with interest on what the team is trying to achieve. Part of contextual thinking, which you learned about in Chapter 3, is associated with work and practice ethic, getting the job done in a professional, effective and efficient manner.

If you have received critical commentary as regards your attitudes or values, I recommend the following:

- Clarify what, specifically, the assessor is referring to, without challenging the assessment itself: 'Can you help me with that point? I need to understand which colleagues I have seemed dismissive of.'
- Ask how the assessment was made. It is unusual for an assessor to reach this judgement by themselves, so ask whether they have conferred with others before reaching the judgement. A professional assessor will usually have conferred on such matters, realising how challenging such an evaluation can seem.
- Ask whether you demonstrated any positive behaviour, that which seemed to convey a better impression of your attitudes and values. It is quite reasonable to ask for assurance that the balance of your behaviour has been considered too.
- Take the criticism away and think about it before raising your concerns with your practice supervisor or link tutor. If you wish to raise points about these matters, write them down and acknowledge both strengths and weaknesses in your practice. Confronting assessors with the challenge 'You're all wrong!' is unconvincing and suggests a lack of insight.

Chapter summary

There are several key messages in this chapter. Learning in clinical practice is different to the explorative and risk-free enquiry of campus, sometimes intense, and you must be an active and organised learner. You help to shape the learning experience by working with your supervisor. But learning in this setting need not seem chaotic. If you approach the placement well organised and ready to study that which you observe, using questions such as those I suggest, there is every chance that you will extract important insights from your placement. Not only will you discover what counts as a problem, how solutions are negotiated, but you will learn a good deal about clinicians and their reasoning templates. You will learn a great deal about healthcare systems and how service is conceived.

Remember that while we learn about person-centred care and work to individualise care, pressures of time and finite resources dictate that care teams must also search for commonly occurring problems and solutions that seem to be beneficial for most patients. These considerations will inform the templates of care as well. A practice template is not something that remains rigid; it is a base from which the nurse can start. Frequently then nurses identify how care needs to be refined for individual patient circumstances.

In clinical practice, you learn about teamwork and professional etiquette. You are socialised to a healthcare system that strives to personalise care wherever possible, but which also must make the most efficient use of finite resources. Clinicians work with imperfect knowledge (e.g. before diagnosis of an illness). Because you need to understand how the team proceeds, the practice supervisor is an important guide.

You need to carefully consider the feedback you receive. It can seem bruising to face criticism about something you thought you were good at; but remember that contexts change, and what worked in one place might not be appropriate in another. Nursing is a profession that works within contexts. The feedback will usually be carefully considered and supported afterwards with a review of what might improve matters.

Activities: brief outline answers

Activity 6.1 Evaluation (page 92)

I think that there is a broad correlation between the learning work that Sue and Phillip describe and the questions what, so what and what next? We must begin by mapping what is going on in the clinical area and that applies to care service as much as individual care episodes. Healthcare teams develop a sense of what they are working collectively towards and the best means to do that. So, we start with the 'what?' of care work. After that Sue and Phillip agree that attention shifts to the clientele and what they have in common. Some problems may occur repeatedly, some needs are commonplace, so as part of the 'so what?' questioning it makes sense to focus on the care to be negotiated and what seems most likely to reassure a range of patients in this setting. 'What next?' questioning then focuses on care solutions, skills and treatment protocols that make a difference. We start to learn about what the healthcare team thinks is effective, welcome and realistic. In practice we begin to uncover the templates that they use to arrange the care service.

This might seem quite startling to you, given that some campus-based teaching centres on individualised care and a nurse-patient one-to-one negotiation. In reality, groups of patients are often nursed, and what is learned about and from groups (problems shared) can materially help the nurse nego-tiate care with individual patients. Our templates about what most patients need or benefit from become the opening speculations about what might aid the individual patient beyond that.

Activity 6.2   Reflection (page 94)

When you join a practice placement, I think that you establish what the nature of work is there and how nurses go about what they do. If you then link this to the knowledge that nurses use and the skills that they deploy you quite quickly identify practice templates. Nurses, for instance, develop a collection of important things to do if patient rehabilitation is the nature of the work conducted. They do much the same if they are managing pain or exploring anxiety and depression. The templates typically include elements of evidence, experience, clinical protocol or legal or ethical requirements and insights offered by the patient or relative themselves. Practice templates are powerful precisely because they operate with the resources of service, the system in which care is made available. Templates are cognisant of financial resources, skills available and the expectations of patients and relatives in commonly recurring situations. They may or may not have been formulated into written care plans, something that could seem rather formulaic (see Useful Websites in this chapter).

It is against this practice environment that we can explore the placement objectives of the module and your skill aspirations. In practice placements there may come times when you deduce that work lags behind best practice, that which evidence offers. On other occasions you may be equipped with searching questions to pose to the philosophy of nursing. Opportunities build for you to develop what Sue described as a utility narrative of care, that worthy of discussion within your portfolio.

Further reading

Hashemiparast, M, Negarandeh, R and Theofanidis, D (2019) Exploring the barriers of utilizing theoretical knowledge in clinical settings: a qualitative study. *International Journal of Nursing Sciences*, 6(4): 399–405.

The authors catalogue a range of confidence issues relating to using theory in practice. Equally significant (I think) is the unwritten assumption that theory is fit for purpose. It is worth speculating on the relative roles of theory and practice. Does theory serve practice or does it direct practice? Is theory born out of practice need or from another place, perhaps professional philosophy?

Standing, M (2023) *Clinical judgement and decision making in nursing*, 5th edition. London: Sage/Learning Matters.

This valuable book leads the reader through different ways of thinking about clinical decision-making and explains how an understanding of ethics, reflection and priorities can lead to better decision-making. Of all the things that can seem mysterious and awe-inspiring in practice, it is the decision-making of experienced practitioners that is the most significant. Reading about these processes is therefore a valuable adjunct to clinical placement learning.

Useful websites

www.birdie.careblog.examples-of-person-centred-care

Birdie (2022) Care plan templates: examples of person-centred care.

A number of commercial organisations have argued that core elements of care planning can be relatively standardised. The argument is made that using template care plans (those offered by the company) sets clearer standards by which care can be judged and helps multidisciplinary care teams to work to common purpose. This web resource takes you to just one offering of this kind.

The question arises though whether care should be a) individually negotiated on every occasion (an ideal of person-centred care), b) whether templates should be generated locally, reflecting local clientele and resources or c) whether commercial companies have something to offer with templates such as offered here. The third option might appeal where administrative work seems onerous, but the counterargument is that care is then inflexible and unresponsive. So, as you complete your placement, I think it's worth pondering just where practice templates usefully come from and how such reasoning might best acknowledge the individuality of patients? If you believe that template reasoning risks inflexible thinking, then that poses very significant reflection in practice work for the nurse. If you accept (as I do) that the development of viable local working templates of care is necessary (that which usually assists patients), then another question arises, how do we counter the risk of formulaic thinking?

Thinking about templates is especially important as you contemplate the relationship between theory and practice, as you find compromises between what each teaches you and as you later deliberate on how best to sustain nursing work over a lifelong career.

Chapter 7 Making use of electronic media

NMC Future Nurse: Standards of Proficiency for Registered Nurses

Because the subject matter covered by electronic media varies widely, there are no specific standards to link to. The skills covered in this chapter underpin how you successfully learn and achieve all of the standards within the environment of electronic media.

Chapter aims

After reading this chapter, you will be able to:

- summarise the ways in which electronic media communication influences critical thinking;
- explore personal interests regarding the use of electronic media in support of learning;
- identify ways in which tutors provide feedback on assignments and how this could be used;
- prepare appropriate contributions to electronic forums associated with your course of studies;
- explore whether a strategic use of electronic resource information might help you marshal your studies and make sense of diverse information.

Introduction

In the last chapter we explored how the practice environment provided opportunities for learning and helped to shape how you understood nursing. We examined the opportunities there to uncover the practice templates that nurses use to deliver care. The electronic resources that you use on your course are no less an environment and they, too, can help you understand nursing and care (e.g. Kirkpatrick, 2020; Mahotra and Kumar, 2021). You might explore patient experiences of illness and care using video or podcast recordings. These offer a rapid overview of common patient concerns and needs as well as how they self-care. But you might also explore what it feels like to consult with others in the analysis of healthcare problems. The work that you do on electronic forums mimic professional healthcare consultation beyond. Imagine, for instance, joining a national forum on the best ways to counter the rapid expansion of a new viral threat. There are circumstances where consultation happens at arm's length, where you cannot see a colleague in the room.

Here are some further benefits of electronic media for your learning:

- Recorded lectures and skill demonstrations can be run online, enabling you to pause and rerun video clips so that you can check over the points made.
- Interactive study online (e.g. electronic forums) acquaints you with technology something that patients may use too. Technology is transforming what it means to be a healthcare consumer (Marx and Padmanabhan, 2020).
- Electronic resources significantly increase your access to knowledge, both within the library through websites, and beyond (Jankowski, 2016; Shakeel and Bhatti, 2018).
- Your study notes, portfolio, and course or placement reports can be stored electronically using a cloud facility. At its simplest, this means carrying around less bulky notebooks and folders.

Activity 7.1   Critical enquiry

Imagine now you are building your understanding of a practice template called 'managing chronic pain'. Remember templates help us frame our approach to care and negotiations with patients, but they are not rigid prescriptions. The template helps you to orientate questions that you might ask the patient, what you might suggest. Go to YouTube (www. youtube.com) and type in the search term 'chronic pain'.

- What sorts of resources did you find there and how might these add to your understanding of how we might usefully counter chronic pain?
- What sort of information was available there? Did it, for instance, centre on patient insights? Was there an emphasis on patient coping? Did you find material on the altered physiology of pain?
- How were patients using pain relief measures?

As you build a practice template you mix and match valuable information including patient testimony such as this, but you will need to carefully evaluate claims made as well.

I will return with answers to this activity as part of Case study 3.

Electronic media has limits too, however. Nursing is a very interpersonal profession, and we also need to engage with people face to face (Stein-Parbury, 2021). Electronic media struggles to simulate the conditions of healthcare practice. Face-to-face role play, for instance, is arguably better than electronic discussion. Interacting online with study group peers in a forum is a different psychological experience to a clinical team meeting. In a team meeting, the words you share in a discussion are said and gone. In an interactive online discussion, they are often typed in or audio-recorded, which can leave you feeling a little more exposed to scrutiny by others: 'I wish I hadn't said that!'

Activity 7.2   Reflection

Pause now to reflect on how you view technology-based learning. If we divide electronic resources into those that deliver information (e.g. library texts, recorded lectures) and those that require interaction on your part (e.g. an electronic forum), which seems the more exciting or useful, and which seems the more challenging?

My answers to this activity are given at the end of the chapter.

In this chapter, we examine what is involved in learning using different electronic media, and I make suggestions about how you can derive benefit from them. To help you link electronic resources to critical thinking I use four case studies: making best use of critical feedback, speculating with colleagues in an electronic forum, working with an electronic classroom and formulating templates for patient care. Let us begin though with a brief description of some resources.

E-mail

Within your nursing course, it is likely that you will be linked to a course web page within the university and have an e-mail account set up for you so that you can communicate with your tutor, the library and study group colleagues.

Just as there is etiquette associated with the use of electronic forums ('netiquette'), so there is one associated with the use of e-mail for educational purposes. Beyond the usual caution that to type in CAPITALS is rude (it equates to shouting), there are other, equally important rules associated with what is and is not to be discussed using e-mail. For example, you may discuss a draft piece of coursework with your tutor by e-mail, but to do so with a study buddy is to risk censure. This is because of university rules concerning academic collusion and the need to ensure that work is not plagiarised.

Wikis

You may not have encountered a wiki before, but it can be described simply as an electronic space where individuals make contributions that add to the understanding of a subject (Trocky and Buckley, 2016). Individuals type their entry to the wiki in a text box, check what they have written, and then post it to the wiki space on the course web page. The purpose of a wiki is to add layers of information – extra interpretations of what has been posted as the subject of the wiki. So, for example, a tutor might ask you to build a collective explanation of 'ethical decision making'. In this way, as each student adds a small contribution, an extended explanation of the concept emerges. The wiki remains online as a reference resource for students to draw on later. Wikis sometimes form the basis of a subsequent electronic seminar where you discuss what has been revealed by the information collated.

Activity 7.3   Critical thinking

Imagine that your tutor has set up a wiki for your study group and invited contributions from each of you. All are asked to add something that they have found. It's a place of reported discoveries. How might that feel for you? Does it help that it's simply a case of contributing and reading? I prompt the reflection to help you understand the extent to which you are instinctively a private or a public learner. Wikis can prove a valuable bridge between private learning and electronic group discussion.

As this is your personal reflection, I don't include an answer at the end of the chapter.

Electronic forums

Most courses offer electronic forums, which are places where students and tutors can communicate with one another, either asynchronously (i.e. over time) or synchronously (i.e. at a designated time) (Adams et al., 2015; Bagbhani et al., 2022). Quite often an electronic forum is used to conduct a seminar where you mutually review the articles that you have read. As with wikis, you access the relevant electronic forum using your student identification number and individual password, a process that ensures the relative privacy of discussions within that space. Individual forum discussions are connected to course modules, and postings made there may demonstrate your 'attendance' or even contribute to course marks achieved.

In the forum, a series of individual discussions is initiated (often by the tutor); as each student adds responses of their own, a 'thread' develops. At different points, the tutor may tidy up the thread, editing material to ensure the final record of discussion remains clear to all.

Electronic classrooms

Electronic forums are valuable, especially the asynchronous ones, as you can visit them when it suits you best. Nonetheless, the conversations can seem a little slow or stilted. For this reason, many universities use electronic classrooms. Electronic classrooms are designed to function as tutorials within the online environment, and they offer significant benefits when it comes to managing study time (Singh, 2021). There are no car parking or public transport expenses associated with attending these tutorials, but you will need access to a modern computer that runs the latest software, as well as a headset microphone, so that you can participate successfully.

You join the electronic classroom using a preset web address (a URL) and log in with your student identification number and individual password. What then appears is a whiteboard screen upon which you or your tutor will be able to draw diagrams, make lists and sketch flow charts. Beside the whiteboard screen, there is a series of control features with which you need to acquaint yourself using university training sessions. Commonly, these features include:

- a facility to ask questions or make points (using your microphone);
- the opportunity to vote in debates or in response to tutor questions;
- a facility to view streamed audio/video material;
- the opportunity to visit other web addresses using hyperlinks provided;
- a facility to move to a 'breakout' room where you conduct small group discussions.

Electronic classrooms usually require a little technical preparation (configuring your computer) and *some* discipline (especially in the use of microphones). They can seem unfamiliar, insofar as you do not necessarily see the faces of other students. Against that, however, they provide real-time interactive learning for students who might not be studying on campus.

Case study 1: Making good use of feedback

We come now to the first of the case studies within this chapter. As part of your coursework, it is possible that you will submit both formative assignments (not graded) and summative assignments (those that are grade bearing) electronically to your tutor, as well as receiving your feedback in a similarly paperless way. Electronic submission has the advantage that you can obtain a record of the assignment being submitted on time. One of the other key advantages of an electronically submitted assignment is that the tutor can give you both summary feedback (as an end-of-work commentary) and feedback in the form of textual annotations which you can read as part of an attachment e-mailed back to you (see Figure 7.1).

Figure 7.1 illustrates two forms of feedback on a single paragraph extract from a student's assignment answer. The first is called 'track changes' and is presented here as underlined text that appears within the body of the essay work. In the first instance, track changes have been used to correct the presentation of a reference. The adjustment shows the correct spelling of the author name and queries the date of publication. In the second track change, the tutor provides guidance on both the referencing of the work and the planning of coherent paragraphs. The second form of feedback consists of marginal annotations using the 'comment' feature. ER in this instance stands for 'educational reviewer'.

(Continued)

(Continued)

Children have particular diffiulties expressing pain. Younger ones have a more limited vocabulary to describe the pain and many use general terms like 'tummy' to refer to its location. They don't have a clear sense of time and many struggle to describe the duration of the pain. Macgrath (1989) [MacGrath (1990) in your reference list [ER1]] explains that nurses have to use parents to help interpret the pain. Parents are familiar with the way in which a child expresses themselves and can help determine whether pain may be a problem, for example when the child seems distracted and unable to concentrate on what they are doing [ER2]. Children have just as much pain as the rest of us and it's wrong to assume that they don't feel pain in the same way as adults. [You need a reference here and perhaps to consider making this a separate paragraph. This paragraph is all about the expression of pain and your last point is about the incidence or nature of pain encountered].

Comment [ER1]: Are there more recent references that you could use?

Comment [ER2]: Do you think there are any circumstances when we need to be more cautious about relying upon a parent to help interpret a child's pain? If you are unsure why not look up 'Munchausen by proxy' syndrome?

Figure 7.1 Examples of track changes and margin note commentary feedback

The purpose of feedback

One purpose of feedback is to correct a misapprehension, whether it concerns a reference, a drug calculation or an assertion about ethical care (McCarthy et al., 2018). Corrections are often handled using track changes, with the tutor either deleting something and inserting the correct material or commenting on the deficits. But other feedback may have a more subtle function. Comment ER1 in Figure 7.1 is designed to prompt some further thought and enquiry. Sometimes feedback is more rhetorical and designed to illustrate the way in which the tutor is 'thinking aloud' (ER2). Tutors do not invariably expect you to respond to every remark. On occasions, the marginal commentary is intentionally provocative as well as rhetorical, as in this example: 'Perhaps we are naive to imagine what can be easily assessed. It is bound up with private experiences, memories and fears. I wonder what you think?'

Making sense of feedback

We need, then, to make sense of the tutor's feedback. Does it require a response on my part? However important a coursework mark or grade might seem, the commentary that accompanies your assignment answer is important too. Even if you have achieved a good mark, there is always something more to glean from the commentary provided. You need to ascertain what the tutor thinks you have learned here and what could remain to be achieved. For instance, does the tutor comment on the structure of your essay answer? Does the feedback highlight your ability to argue a case?

Doing something with feedback

While logistically tutors supporting large student groups cannot share protracted dialogue with every student, there is a strong case for corresponding further with your tutor in the following circumstances:

- where you have received a poor grade and/or where the commentary suggests that you have misunderstood the question;
- where the commentary suggests a significant gap in your subject knowledge;
- where the feedback has posed new questions to you (you wish to ask the tutor to help clarify a matter);
- where the tutor has suggested other possible lines of enquiry.

In the above circumstances, tutors really do welcome your follow-up enquiry. The conversations that follow on from the assignment feedback will help you to develop your powers of discrimination and argument formation.

Activity 7.4   Reflection

Reflect now on what if any use you have made of tutor assignment feedback offered to you. If you didn't act on it, have subsequent assignment answers demonstrated similar faults?

As this answer is based on your own reflection, there is no outline answer at the end of the chapter.

Case study 2: Speculating with others in the forum

My second case example of electronic media-mediated learning concerns the use of electronic forums. Tutors use these forums for various purposes, including the clarification of values, beliefs and attitudes. Making contributions to the electronic forum can seem more difficult, though. I asked Fatima to reflect on contributing to forums. She said:

> *I have enjoyed the different forums. To read other people's ideas is encouraging. But posting my ideas was more difficult. I dislike conflict, arguing about whose ideas are right!*

Fatima's reflections are familiar to tutors. However, making arguments is necessary if you are to advance your thinking. There is a need to speculate and explore arguments with supportive peers and an empathetic tutor. Happily, the system for posting forum messages involves composition and there is a chance to review your posting before you press 'send'. While most students do this to check their grammar and syntax, the greatest benefit of the pre-submission check is being able to consider whether your points seem clear to you. No one in the forum expects perfection. No one anticipates that their comments will always be supported either. Just as in other conversations, there will be some good points made and some that seem more questionable.

Activity 7.5   Critical thinking

Imagine that you are engaged in a forum discussion about end-of-life care and discussion turns to the patient's 'right' to end life early (voluntary euthanasia). Student A expresses the view that to do this contravenes religious faith values. Student B reflects that legal risks arise if a carer collaborates in such a decision. Student C counters though that dignity of life is important too and patients are best placed to determine what represents quality of life at this stage. How might you contribute next to this shared speculation? Jot down your ideas before turning to my next points.

In Chapter 1, you were introduced to the business of making arguments. But real-time electronic forums are often difficult places to make formal arguments. We are after all thinking on our feet. One of the reasons that Fatima might find it uncomfortable offering responses in an electronic forum could be that she thinks her offerings are 'just ideas'. Ideas, those speculated upon are important though. Oftentimes we creep up on better explanations of what is happening through discussion.

In the discussion (Activity 7.5) student A offers a speculation about others' rights as well as those of the patient. Nurses have rights as well, those linked to deeply held religious convictions, but you might respond that these need to be recognised and consulted upon well in advance (Allen, 2022). It's less professional to reveal them in retrospect if the nurses practised in a setting where end-of-life care was a regular part of the work. You are not confronting student A and saying, 'you're wrong!', you are suggesting that with rights come responsibilities too.

Student B offers a factual point; the law (in whichever land you practise) takes a position on voluntary euthanasia (Close et al., 2021). Responding to a claimed fact you could say 'but that's not true!'; facts are open to clarification and dispute. But you could also reflect on whether the law is clear in every regard?

Student C expresses a value (Maio, 2016), asserting that if we are being adequately person centred then the patient should have a significant say in such a matter. It's this speculation that offers extensive scope for discussion because it's centre stage in the euthanasia debate. You might think 'goodness, where do I start!', but remember that the forum often isn't a place of absolute truth, it's a place of clearer understanding. Your individual response doesn't have to solve the problem.

What can we say, then, about the business of contributing within electronic forums? First, it seems necessary to accept that forums are not the same as face-to-face seminars. They leave a record, so you will naturally wish to compose your contributions carefully. Second, successful forums are permissive and allow that arguments might develop within and through them. You will make several observations and the clarity of matters will improve as the group takes stock of what has been posted. It is OK to 'feel your way' in these matters. Your tutor has a key role here, helping to sum up points. Third, discussions held in electronic forums are not and should not be reputation busters. Your tutor should make this clear at the outset; otherwise, trust will not grow within the study group.

Case study 3: Interacting successfully within the electronic classroom

In the third case study, we turn to successful learning within the electronic classroom. Although you have already learned valuable principles while reading about learning from lectures (Chapter 4) and seminars (Chapter 5), there are some subtle variations here that you need to be aware of. Much of what you need to consider now relates to attending sensitively to the needs of fellow learners, as well as making the technology work for everyone. As you cannot necessarily see other class participants, you must imagine how they feel as they interface with the classroom using a computer.

Preparation begins before the class itself; you should ensure that you approach discussion inquisitively. Note on what date and at what time the session begins. It can be very disruptive to join the class late and then try to catch up on what has already been done. To ensure that you can contribute fully, complete a brief computer check. Most of the electronic classroom platforms have a log-on wizard facility, which allows you to check that you can hear the audio output clearly and test that your microphone is working well. Familiarise yourself with the various control functions at your command within the electronic classroom. Check to see that you can turn your microphone on and off (the screen icon will change). You need to have your microphone off when you are not speaking, otherwise your open-channel microphone might block a fellow student.

The classroom is likely to have a separate response box where you can type in text (e.g. a question). Conduct a trial run before the class to ensure that your typed text appears in the box as expected. Your tutor will be able to see this while running the session. Do not assume, however, that all student queries are instantly acted on. Responses may be saved for a summing-up point. Identify whether you may indicate your understanding of the session using emoticons (smiling or frowning faces). Your tutor might rely on these to determine the pace and direction that the class takes.

Attending to the class itself requires a little extra thought as well. Remember that you will be seated before a computer screen, possibly many miles from the university itself. So, I recommend that you:

* have a notebook and pencil to hand (you may wish to compose queries or reflections carefully before posting these within the electronic classroom);
* have refreshments to hand (avoid spilling liquids on the computer, however);
* use the 'out of the room' icon to indicate when you are not present in class.

(Continued)

(Continued)

Class sizes vary, but a key consideration is to post responses, either typed or audio, that seem constructive. Remember that you cannot see the scowls of other students in this environment. So, monitor whether others have already typed in questions or reflections within the text box, and where possible save your points for the frequent 'Are you all happy?' breaks that experienced tutors tend to use. If you wish to refer to something specifically, note down the location in your notebook: 'I have a query about slide 4 in your presentation.'

Where students agree, classroom sessions are archived (i.e. they are recorded) so that you and your fellow students can access them again later. If this has not been agreed, however, you will need to make notes as you proceed through the class. PowerPoint presentations are often sent to you by the tutor for later reference. Anticipate, however, that at the end of the session, you may be asked to conclude what you understood. Having notes to hand will help you to do that and to indicate what you hope to follow up study on. As with face-to-face lectures, the notes made here are likely to be brief and will need expansion after the class has finished.

Case study 4: Building a practice template

Over the pages of this book, you have been learning about templates that both help you understand nursing and help fashion our approach to individual patients. The purpose of practice templates is to help us negotiate care when you are already conversant with common patient experiences and needs, relevant evidence, policies and protocols (Buchanan et al., 2021). Electronic resources can substantially assist you as you work on chosen templates that you think might be important to a wide range of patients and which facilitate cost effective study for you. To illustrate this work, we will return to the management of chronic pain, that which you met in Activity 7.1.

Table 7.1 summarises the electronic source materials that could assist you to build a template for the managing of chronic pain in patients.

Practice templates are where various elements of your study come together. They lead us through the 'what', the 'so what' and to the 'what next' questions important in practice (Rolfe et al., 2011). At first, gathering and collating so much information from different sources might seem daunting, but it's worth remembering that such templates might materially assist you with individual module assessments and they can run incrementally across several modules of study. Chronic pain is important in a variety of nursing fields of work and in different care settings. Exploring a practice template can be an enquiry that you initiate, which offers focus to your portfolio of studies (see Chapter 12), and which increases your confidence as you meet new patients in later clinical placements. Exploring practice templates can prove motivating and exciting and might in the longer term even lead to specialisation within your nursing career.

Electronic resource	Notes
Video and podcast patient testimony about the experience of chronic pain and the use of different treatments to counter it.	This material offers you 'broad scope' summary of how pain is interpreted, what is most distressing and how coping is conceived. You will still explore individual needs when negotiating care, but this information assists you to enquire with purpose about what *might* be needed.
Recorded lectures on the theory of pain and its management, the philosophy and ethics of pain management in different contexts such as end-of-life care.	Theory models a phenomenon like pain, explaining key arguments about controlling rather than countering pain in retrospect.
Website material on available treatment modalities, the benefits, and the limits of different medications.	We need to learn about the available tools at our disposal. These are not without controversy as different treatment modalities have their advocates.
Electronic journals and textbooks reporting research on assessment and management of chronic pain, and patient response to the same.	Some of the above source material could become dated, so we need to understand new horizons ideas, that which might improve the care offer to patients.
Case study-based seminars where colleagues describe work to help patients manage chronic pain.	Case studies illustrate how problems can be unique or contextual and they illustrate how different elements of care are sometimes combined.
Portfolio reflections on practical pain management gleaned from practice placements.	We secure first-hand accounts of what seems to work, what might be problematic when managing chronic pain. We are reminded about caveats to more formulaic care.
Electronic records of codes, protocols and policies	We are reminded of the service and the professional standards context, that which balances individual care negotiation.

Table 7.1 Building a practice template using electronic resources (manachronic pain)

To build a practice template though, you will need to:

- develop search skills, in the library and beyond;
- critically examine information found;
- weigh the importance of different information, particularly with regard to what is realisable within practice, what is ethical and acceptable to patients;
- determine how you might summarise your reasoning to patients, lay carers and professional colleagues.

In previous decades, and without the benefit of such rich and diverse, readily accessible electronic information it was harder for nurses to comprehensively identify better ways to practice. Nurses were locked in debates about what should be done, some arguing for the

(Continued)

(Continued)

preeminence of clinical experience, others for the importance of research evidence and yet others the need to negotiate as much care as possible with individual patients (Butts and Rich, 2021). Now there is an opportunity to build and discuss practice templates. Nurses cannot realistically negotiate all care from scratch at each new care encounter. There is a need to draw strategically upon what has already been discovered regarding other patients' experiences.

In association with Activity 7.1 I conducted my own review of video and podcast information relating to chronic pain and its management. It was important to move cautiously as not only might source material be dated, but it could be presented in a biased way. For instance, there are fervent advocates of non-medication pain management approaches and competing advocates who favour pharmacy solutions. As I explored resources upon the internet, I had to remind myself of the need to determine who authored material and which organisations they represented. Chapter 8 details the need to bring a quizzical eye to research evidence and you need to be no less critical when evaluating web material. One of the things I realised is that a practice template demands that we make decisions about which information is the most authoritative (influential or powerful), which is the most authentic (relating to patient needs) and which is most realisable (conceding that resources are not infinite). Authoritative information (for example large-scale, well-designed research evidence) might offer clear benefits but if these were in nature difficult for patients and their lifestyles, the chances of practice change were reduced. A practice template focuses upon that which is realisable as well as desirable.

Focusing in upon my discoveries among the testimonial material I identified several points that seemed relevant to how I might approach a patient suffering from chronic pain. I illustrate these with some YouTube video clips. Set aside the therapy/organisational promotional elements of these and concentrate on the patient narrative. My points included the following:

- Pain is frequently referenced against lifestyle and what the individual normally does. It's not a concept that stands apart from the patient's life. The extent to which a patient perseveres coping with pain is often influenced by their sense of social responsibility. It is then unwise to ask simply about the location, intensity and frequency of pain; I need to ask about daily living too. It is this which might help motivate or sustain the patient.

  o Take a look at Linda Wilhelm's experience of coping with arthritic pain, searching for treatment options that work within her lifestyle, Canadian Arthritis Patient Alliance, **https://youtu.be/R45t_vRslCc?feature=shared**

- Patients habitually describe their chronic pain using analogies, images that they hope that the clinician can relate to, and which might elicit support. While such images are not necessarily actionable (turned into a therapy or a treatment), we need to listen attentively to them to build rapport with the patient. This is especially true with chronic pain that does not have a clear trauma onset and where patients may fear that we doubt them.

o   Take a look at 'Fibromyalgia; living with chronic pain' from BBC Stories. **https://youtu.be/1CBULIcf9MU**

- Pain has far-reaching effects, forcing the patient to revisit their notion of self and social worth amongst others. Pain has to be negotiated with others, its impact explained to those who investigate it.

o   Take a look at 'Struggling with pain', an actor-presented account of one woman's chronic but frustratingly ambiguous back pain. You will find it **at https://youtu.be/FPpu7dXJFRI?feature=shared.**

- Patients rarely sit still and simply tolerate their pain; they embark on a journey to explain it to themselves and others. Patients dealing with chronic pain may become experts regarding the origins of their pain and associated illness. While medication might help reduce pain, listening to the account is equally important, reducing a sense of isolation.

o   Take a look at 'Marqus v.'s vhronic pain story' US Pain Foundation Inc. **https://youtu.be/VG-T4pPIWA8**. Marqus deals with a physical crisis pain but also the threat of progressive damage to his body.

Accounts such as the above are important in any template understanding of chronic pain. They signal what seems most important to patients and they may help counter the feeling that we have limited resources to treat chronic pain. When we later combine a review of such video tape or podcast patient accounts, with research evidence, theory insights and ethical best practice principles, we are likely to be in a more confident position to offer care to the patient. Using a mix of electronic resources we might secure a more rounded understanding of care requirements.

Activity 7.6   Reflection

Template exploration centres on that which may be beneficial and realisable. Does the emphasis seem important? If you have worried about a theory-practice gap in your education, does this focus empower you to judge what you will rate most important in your education? If you explore one or more practice templates (those applicable to a range of patients), do you think that this might build confidence as you later start work as a registered nurse? Finally, if studies feel scattered, drawing you in different directions does the exploration of templates, through rich electronic media resources, bring order to your studies, or does it simply seem a daunting project?

As this answer is based on your own observation, there is no outline answer at the end of the chapter.

Chapter summary

In this chapter, I began with the argument that electronic media has much to offer learning, but some careful thought is required when using it. The way you reason using electronic media will be different from reasoning in class. This is not to suggest, however, that these media in some way undermine the critical thinking and reflection that can operate here. The quality of feedback possible with an electronically submitted assignment, the excitement that can be generated in an electronic classroom, the richness of information on the internet, and the depth of debate possible within an electronic forum can be exceptional. The very fact that you can access conversations at times to suit you, and that there is space to compose your answers with care that is not available in a real-time face-to-face conversation, highlights the critical thinking opportunities here.

Electronic media is not without challenges though, and you may have observed within this chapter just how different this communication can seem. For some, it feels artificial, especially if students are private and contemplative in nature. If electronic learning environments are poorly designed, the reputation of electronic learning quickly deteriorates. It is at its best where the tutor introduces fascinating resources to which the class has prompt access, which then form the focus of attention for discussion. It is at its best where tutors help students to direct and shape their enquiries when exploring electronic resources well beyond the campus itself. The electronic learning environment works at different levels, from a discrete discussion upon a submitted essay, right up to a practice template investigation that might span several modules of study.

Activities: brief outline answers

Activity 7.2   Reflection (page 105)

My doctoral research was upon the ways in which students conceived learning and negotiated tutor support. Some saw learning as receiving large amounts of information, that interpreted and evaluated by academic staff. In short, students hoped that tutors might convey the truth of a subject. Other learners were much more inquisitive and positively enjoyed the ambiguity of knowledge, accepting that learning (in effect) never ended. I learned that there was often a correlation between those who wished to learn privately and who preferred more definitive teaching of a subject (truth delivered). Students who were more orientated towards public learning online (shared discovery) were usually more comfortable with the ambiguity of knowledge. Indeed, this second group of learners doubted that there was an absolute truth to be discovered in many areas of the syllabus.

I suspect that our preference for either private or public learning, taught resources or shared enquiry, are a function of our past education and confidence levels. It may too be linked to whether we habitually process information slowly and cautiously or whether we like to 'explore and see'. Both preferences have something to commend them, but it remains the case that nursing does require collaboration and sometimes, action before we have marshalled every piece of information. It's important then to gently stretch and challenge your learning preferences, so that you remain adaptable.

Electronic resources provide opportunity for both preferred learning approaches. Private enquiries are possible using the internet and the library, those guided by your tutor but those which excite you as well. Within the electronic forums of the module there is scope, too, for collaboration and debate.

Further reading

Flyverbom, M (2019) *The digital prism: transparency and managed visibilities in a datafied world.* Cambridge: Cambridge University Press.

Mikkel Flyverbom reminds us that digital technology is increasingly intruding into every aspect of modern life, sometimes obtrusively so. The argument runs that the digital revolution increases connectivity between people but diminishes privacy. It is well worth thinking about, for instance, with regard to patient records and the safety and reputation of healthcare professionals. Is there a case to limit such technology, and if so when is that point reached?

Shackleton-Jones, N (2023) *How people learn: a new model of learning and cognition to improve performance and education,* 2nd edition. Kogan Page: London.

I spend some time every year talking with students who admit that their nursing course seems alien to them. It is not that they cannot understand the subject matter taught, it is that the learning projects and activities required of them seem quite at odds with how they reason. In some instances, this problem might be linked to poor module design, a strategy inadequately explained. In others though it is because the learner has never paused to consider how they prefer to reason, which ways it seems easiest to think. This book then is a resource for you the student in difficulty or for academic staff designing new modules. While it doesn't spend a great deal of time reviewing learning in the electronic environment (and it's not focused on nursing), it should help you understand where difficulties might be arising with your enquiries and coursework. We have touched on private versus public learning here, but Nick Shackleton-Jones explores a range of difficulties beyond.

Useful websites

I want to suggest two useful resources found on YouTube (**www.youtube.com**).

The first is for any of you who feel lost by the multitude of information available on the internet, entitled *How I learn things online (way more efficiently)* by Nathaniel Drew (**www.youtube.com/watch?v=rVmMbMa3ncI**). Nathaniel is a photographer and an enthusiastic speaker on the personal organisation of enquiry. You will have access to dedicated university library resources, but it is still valuable to contemplate what the internet offers. If you venture there, then your enquiries will need to be disciplined. Nathaniel researches photography, but his enquiry principles still hold good for healthcare.

The second resource is entitled *How to use Zoom for remote and online learning* by Flipped Classroom Tutorials (**www.youtube.com/watch?v=9guqRELB4dg**). Universities use a variety of platforms to deliver online classroom teaching, and this is just one of them. What it does do, however, is to help you understand how the tutor manages such an environment. There is no reason why a group of nurses cannot band together to use such a platform for professional update purposes. Sue (our case study registered nurse) helps to run a journal club using this technology. Each takes a turn running the monthly meetings and every session reviews at least one research article.

Part 3   Expressing critical thought and reflection

Chapter 8　Critiquing evidence-based literature

Chapter aims

After reading this chapter, you will be able to:

- outline the different ways in which evidence might be defined;
- referring to paradigms, summarise why evidence needs to be analysed in different ways;
- discuss validity, reliability, transferability and authenticity as key criteria by which to examine evidence;
- use insights from the ongoing debates about better research evidence to explain why the application of knowledge to practice is not always easy.

Introduction

In a healthcare world where there is an increasing amount of information, theory and evidence, two overarching questions should exercise our thinking. The first is: To what extent are theory and evidence applicable in practice? This is an important question to consider because not all information is realistically utilisable in healthcare. Some philosophical material, for example, is designed to help conceptualise what nursing might be like (Nelson-Brantley et al., 2019). Person-centred care writers make recommendations for practice but might concede that only a percentage of the ideal practice is possible now. For person-centred care to work entirely, not only must healthcare be amply resourced, but it would have to operate with patients ready to partner nurses in care (Price, 2022). If we do not ask questions about the utility of information for practice, we risk cognitive dissonance (Corcoran and Cook, 2023).

The second and more discrete question concerns the nature of evidence and how we can best evaluate it. We think of evidence as a superior kind of information, although it, too, has limits (Jolly, 2020). If evidence were all of one kind, then our evaluative work would be much easier. We would simply work with a series of universal questions to check whether the evidence is sound. In this chapter, though, you will discover that evidence is not all of one kind and that there are then different questions to be asked about each of these.

The importance of utility

Periodically within this book, I have encouraged you to ask whether ideas are realisable in practice. This is not to simply promote cynicism; it is instead to acknowledge limits to the uses that particular information can reasonably be put. Let me illustrate. In the 1990s, I developed a theory of body image to help nurses understand how patients dealing with a wide variety of injuries and illnesses might experience their bodies as damaged (Price, 1990). The implication was that if we could understand patient distress then we could develop supportive measures to help them cope.

The simple triangular model describing how body image is experienced proved very successful. It was a useful explanatory device. But the theory of altered body image care (what came next) proved harder to action. This was because it assumed some counselling ability of the nurse, adequate time to explore the experience, and recognition that body image care had to be shared across different agencies. Nurses in hospitals often referred patients on to others in the community. An acutely distressed patient might need the help of a psychologist. The key point was that my theory had value but also limits. Body image care was often therapy, and debates then arose about how to ensure its continuity.

I share this illustration to emphasise that information shared in many areas of nursing is a work in progress. Something that started as a means of explaining a phenomenon (altered body image) began to expand into a guide on how to practise to best effect.

The problem was that the theory had finite utility. However compelling it was profession-ally, it was limited by issues associated with healthcare resources and by practitioner skills.

As you discuss theory and research evidence on campus, there are a series of questions that you can use to check the practice utility of what is promoted. In the event that you conclude the information has finite practice utility, it may still have purpose elsewhere. For example, the information may inform the professional philosophy of nursing. Just because information is difficult to utilise now does not mean that it does not have professional merit.

Here are the suggested questions:

- *What assumptions are made about patients and their next of kin?* Care is fundamentally a collaborative activity. We proceed with the patient's insight and informed consent, so this becomes an acid test of what theory or evidence can be used with confidence in practice.
- *What assumptions are made about the role of the nurse and their skills?* Some of the theory and evidence that you meet on campus might only be within the remit and the skill set of an advanced practitioner or consultant nurse. Other information might be usable by a range of nurses.
- *What assumptions are made about the range and appropriate focus of a healthcare service?* This is quite tricky as in some regards service provision might be confused. Different agencies might do different things, and different hospitals might work with different protocols. Nevertheless, the question is an important one.
- *What assumptions are made about interprofessional working?* The remit of nursing has expanded in recent decades, but there remains role overlap and gaps that can make care decision-making, consultation and collaboration more difficult (Lee et al., 2023).

Activity 8.1   Reflection

Each of the four questions above relate to whether nursing care can really be homogenous (that is, much the same everywhere). Given your experience of clinical placements just how var-ied does nursing practice seem? How context specific is the research that you have read to date?

I offer a brief reflection at the end of the chapter.

The nature of evidence

We can turn now to the second question and the nature of evidence. To explore this subject, I return to the four case study nursing students who we first met in Chapter 1. Each has searched for and engaged with evidence within the healthcare literature. But as we shall see below, critical thinking – when it is applied to evidence – is not straight-forward. Evidence is neither a neutral nor a straightforward concept, and the way in which evidence is defined may influence how it is then evaluated.

Activity 8.2   Critical thinking

Below I set out the opening definitions of evidence that Stewart, Fatima, Raymet and Gina have used to search for information. I asked them to illustrate their points, referring to the topic of pain and its management. As you can see, they are quite different, and as a result different sorts of literature might be found.

Decide which of the following definitions of evidence seem most convincing to you.

As this answer is based on your own observation, there is no outline answer at the end of the chapter.

Case study: Four definitions of 'evidence'

Gina: I've always thought of evidence as that which science, and in particular experimental research or randomised controlled trials, produces. What distinguishes evidence from mere information is that the knowledge has been secured by design; there is a rigorous method to the work, and we can evaluate that. So, for me, there is an emphasis on pain interventions, medication and other treatments that might make a discernible difference.

Fatima: Maybe! But you're missing something here – evidence isn't restricted to research. Audits, patient satisfaction surveys, case studies of unusual patient situations and needs, what we did to look after them, that counts as evidence too. Pain is individual, so we need a wide-ranging appreciation of it.

Raymet: So what about the evidence of your own eyes, then? If reflection doesn't produce a sort of evidence too, aren't we missing out on something? Not everything can be examined in a piece of research. Nurses accumulate insights into pain, the emotional as well as the physical sort, and that needs to be considered too.

Stewart: Perhaps, then, evidence is that which you can measure, that which you can quantify. Other sorts of information are still important, but we shouldn't try to make evidence stretch so far, to serve every situation. We need evidence and patient stories – their narratives about coping with pain. Evidence, though, that should be apolitical, shouldn't it? It should be produced by those who don't have a particular axe to grind about healthcare and how care should be.

It might not surprise you to learn that evidence has been defined in all of the above ways, from either something quite distinct from other classes of knowledge to something that embraces a wide range of experience and insight (Ellis, 2020). Here, I suggest that evidence might be considered to be information that for the individual, group or organisation has greater authority than some other forms of knowledge, but which still requires scrutiny before it can be appropriately used.

Debates about what represents best evidence are not always solely about judging how the evidence has been secured. They are sometimes about what knowledge nurses should use, as well as what should be the proper study and the basis of nursing practice. If we research human experiences (e.g. that of the patient), then we may produce evidence that can tell us things about how nursing might be experienced, but we might not be able to predict outcomes for large groups of patients.

When the world-famous Cochrane Library was set up (www.cochranelibrary.com), it focused firmly upon a quite discrete form of evidence, concerned with interventions and cause-and-effect relationships. It focused upon treatments and what might be proven to work. Subsequently, the Cochrane Library has considered a rather more wide-ranging collection of evidence, which relates to experiences in healthcare as well. It has been accepted that evidence in healthcare needs to relate to different things, not only interventions, but analysis of experiences, problems, perceptions and preferences as well. The need to diversify the understanding of 'evidence' has grown as nurses and others have become increasingly concerned with healthcare quality, and quality has been understood in experiential as well as effectiveness terms (Linsley and Kane, 2022).

I argue that evidence can only be critically evaluated when: (a) the original premises of the research or other knowledge are understood; and (b) we understand the conventions for critiquing that particular sort of evidence. You need to consider what your own attitude towards knowledge is, what is considered least and most important, and what you support as an essential resource upon which to draw when advancing nursing care (see Figure 8.1).

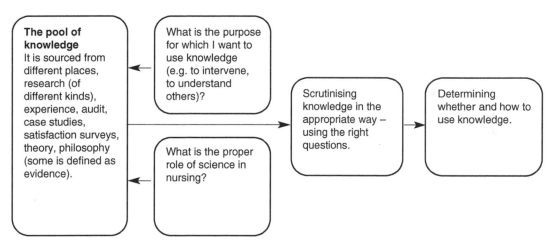

Figure 8.1   Approaching knowledge

Knowledge and how to know it

Thomas Kuhn's classic 1962 book *The Structure of Scientific Revolutions*, one of the most influential philosophy texts of the last century, continues to exercise philosophers (Hedesan and Tendeler, 2017). Kuhn was eager to explain that there could be quite sudden and sometimes violent shifts in thinking, as well as what was accepted as truth. What represented incontrovertible evidence was, as it were, 'up for grabs'. One established way of understanding the world and conducting science therein (we call it a paradigm) could be disputed and replaced by another. The positivist paradigm centres upon the empirical world, that which can be manipulated and tested, and can be controlled – or at least managed – within laboratory and (to a lesser degree) clinical settings. The positivist paradigm draws heavily upon research methods associated with the natural sciences, and work concentrates on trying to demonstrate and measure cause-and-effect relationships, the limiting of researcher bias, and the testing of hypotheses (prediction of what would or would not be the case). Positivist science is classically associated with three things: accurate mapping, precise measurement and strategic manipulation (Ariel et al., 2021). There is often an emphasis upon statistical data, so that it is sometimes called 'quantitative research', although numerical data alone inadequately captures the philosophical premises of such research. Well-designed positivist surveys map phenomena (e.g. anxiety traits) while experimental designs and randomised controlled trials manipulate things (e.g. the dosage of a particular drug given to patients).

Activity 8.3 Reflection

Pause at this stage to reflect upon the implications of the positivist conception of research for nursing. If scientific knowledge comprises what can be manipulated under controlled conditions, how well does this relate to nursing practice?

As this answer is based on your own observation, there is no outline answer at the end of the chapter.

The problem for many nurses was that the positivist paradigm, as well as its conception of knowledge, paid little attention to the practical conditions under which many people lived. The need to design studies that controlled for all undue influences (variables) meant that experiments could be exacting but they might not relate well to practical care situations. Within the healthcare world, there was little chance of controlling all the factors that could influence how individuals behaved, and in any case it was argued that people did not behave according to trait, but – in many instances – according to circumstance. Predicting human behaviour was problematic. As a result of this, a new paradigm or collective world view began to develop and compete with the positivist paradigm. This new world view is sometimes referred to as the naturalistic paradigm because researchers worked in social world conditions with fewer checks and controls on enquiry. The new paradigm is also sometimes referred to as the interpretive paradigm because there was a greater freedom for the researcher to interpret data, especially the experiences of others. Some healthcare research textbooks use the term 'qualitative research' to emphasise the focus on experiences and accounts as data. But whatever we choose to call this new paradigm, it certainly includes a much-increased concern with insights into human experience (Pope and Mays, 2020). The work of the researcher is much less about designing tests and more about enquiring within the social world in an authentic and sensitive fashion (e.g. interviews, observations in practice, case studies).

Activity 8.4   Critical thinking

What do you think the implications are of naturalistic paradigm reasoning for nursing and nursing research? For example, researchers working in this paradigm are very concerned to reveal the different ways in which patients experience the support of the nurse. But because the researcher is less concerned with controlling the data, the evidence resulting from this sort of research is often illustrative – it suggests what could be the case and expects the reader to determine whether their own experience matches what was reported.

As this answer is based on your own observation, there is no outline answer at the end of the chapter.

Debates continue between those who support positivism and those who support naturalism in nursing research (Cresswell and Cresswell, 2018). Arguments are made about what does or does not constitute 'proper science'. The matter is still more complicated, however, by the emergence of a third competing paradigm that also produces research, the critical theory paradigm, which was founded upon the premise that knowledge is rarely neutral (Torres and Nyaga, 2021). Knowledge inherently carries power and there are many people within the world who are eager to use it. Marxist researchers (who challenge class or other political elites) and feminist researchers (who argue that women and other disadvantaged groups are poorly served in society) work within this paradigm. These researchers propose that investigators use research to expose injustices and to empower others to take greater charge of their lives. As a result, a lot of research in this paradigm has been described as action research, consisting of cycles of collaborative activity to improve the lot of disadvantaged groups in healthcare.

Activity 8.5   Critical thinking

What are your reactions to this sort of science, where researchers are engaged in openly political terms, righting perceived wrongs or else empowering others to change the healthcare world?

As this answer is based on your own observation, there is no outline answer at the end of the chapter.

Having formulated your reflections on research paradigms, turn back now to Table 3.1 in Chapter 3. There you will see described different levels of reasoning. Absolute reasoning associated with research paradigms might be to conclude that there is only one sort of 'proper research'. You might fiercely argue this against all comers, but are there any advantages in linking paradigms of research to different contexts and care requirements?

As you think about the different paradigms, it might be tempting to conclude that you should favour a single paradigm. But to back oneself into a philosophical corner might not prove that helpful. Nurses have to work pragmatically and imaginatively with different sorts of knowledge and a range of evidence within healthcare. It is, then, arguably appropriate to adopt a 'horses for courses' attitude towards knowledge. Instead of arguing that one sort of knowledge is superior, it may be appropriate to venture that the key consideration is to what purpose the evidence is put. If we are currently concerned with an intervention and what works, it is likely that we will search for and evaluate knowledge from the positivist paradigm. We will use questions that are appropriate there, which work with the claims of the research (research design and rigour). If we are currently concerned with insights and understanding patients better, we might search for information from the naturalistic paradigm and might ask different questions again. If a convincing case has been made for change, and the improvement involves a shift in power, we might draw on research from the critical theory paradigm and perhaps engage in research ourselves as part of an action research group. The key point is that we think critically in different ways and to strategic purpose. There is no one-size-fits-all way of reasoning possible here.

Asking different questions of evidence

It would be extremely helpful if research authors confided, at the outset, the paradigm within which they have framed their work. In practice, though, this does not always happen. Authors working within the positivist paradigm rarely allude to the philosophy of science that underpins their work, instead moving straight to the design of the survey or experiment. Researchers working within the naturalistic and critical theory paradigms are likely to be more explicit about their philosophical premises, and may refer to a research approach that is clearly aligned to certain beliefs about the nature of knowledge and its role in healthcare. You get a clearer steer as regards the basis on which they are presenting data and findings to you.

Activity 8.6 Group working

To help you to test out my assertions above, arrange with your fellow students to each review a research paper on an agreed theme (something of common interest to you all). Read your chosen paper, highlighting any passages of work that you think indicate the paradigm within which the work was conceived. Clues may be a focus on empirical data, traits, measurement, experimentation and very detailed control measures in the research design, within positivist research. Clues to research conducted within the naturalistic paradigm include reference to research approaches used there, phenomenology, grounded theory, much ethnography, and – quite frequently – case study research. There is an emphasis on natural working environments, discovery and insights into the experience of others. Clues to research conducted within the critical theory paradigm are terms such as 'feminist research' or 'Marxist research', and perhaps the use of 'action research' – work designed to produce rather than investigate change.

Next, summarise your paper to your fellow students, then discuss which paradigm you think it originated from and what that might mean for its contribution to nursing practice.

As this answer is based on your own observation, there is no outline answer at the end of the chapter.

Questions in the positivist paradigm

Where it is concluded that evidence has been produced within the positivist paradigm, a new group of questions becomes important (Aeriel et al., 2021). The first of these relates to the design of the research, and whether it has set out a clear question or hypothesis (a statement regarding what will or will not be the case). The research has to be clearly structured and needs to state precisely which population of people it relates to and what the sample is. The way in which the sample was selected is important in this paradigm because the sample is sometimes argued to represent the population as a whole. The reader has to be convinced that the sample constitutes a reasonable proportion of the population concerned and matches its key features (e.g. age distribution, gender, health circumstances). Statistical guidance is usually sought as regards what represents an adequate sample, and beyond that a satisfactory return rate for questionnaires if a survey is used. Consideration of the population and sample size, the make-up of the sample, and whether it is representative of the population affect study *validity*. The research is valid if it addresses the research intention set and includes relevant and large enough samples of research subjects (people) or clinical circumstances. Small and unrepresentative samples of people can all undermine the validity of the research.

A second concern within positivist paradigm research is *reliability* (Aeriel et al., 2021) – whether, using the same data-gathering methods and the same research design, similar results could be obtained at a later date. Of course, when dealing with human beings, reliability could prove to be a problem. Positivist paradigm research works well where individuals behave or comment according to trait (i.e. consistently, indicative of their stable attitudes and values), but it is less reliable if people change their responses or behaviours dependent on circumstance (e.g. meeting a currently felt need). If people changed their mind frequently and behaved inconsistently, it would be difficult to judge whether the research was reliable.

I asked Stewart to summarise why positivist paradigm researchers were so interested in things such as validity and reliability. This is what he – quite reasonably – said:

Well, the research is about judging something, isn't it? And if you're going to claim that something is or is not proven, then you have to be sure that all your methods are well organised, that the work focuses on exactly the right thing. You have to be sure that others could repeat your work, to check that they got similar results.

A further legitimate question regarding positivist paradigm research is that of bias. Has the researcher in some way, wittingly or otherwise, shaped the evidence so that it is not representative of reality (e.g. by using leading questions)? Has the researcher failed to resist the undue shaping of evidence by people or factors not anticipated in the research? Positivist paradigm researchers are keen to control for bias and to limit the risk that external factors in some way shape the data in ways that undermine subsequent claims about them.

Questions in the naturalistic paradigm

The critical questions to be asked of evidence stemming from the naturalistic paradigm are different and much more about comparing the researcher's account against your own experience of phenomena. This is because the world is conceived of more in terms of perception and experience. Everyone interprets their experiences and creates their own reality – their own account of what is really happening. So, for example, five people may visit the dentist and have treatment, but the experience and the meaning of these visits will depend as much on their perceptions of dentistry. The emphasis here is on the perceptual world, that which is negotiated and even co-created. Think, for example, about the meaning of old age: it is more than a physiological change; it is a complex experience.

Researchers working in this paradigm are not claiming to present a demonstrable truth that can be tested again and again, but a representation of what they have seen, heard and interpreted (Pope and Mays, 2020). Typically, the researcher deals with field observations and open-question interview responses, necessitating the presentation of possible themes, as well as that which might convey what has been experienced. The researcher cannot avoid using their own experiences to help make sense of what was said or witnessed. Because researchers are working with interpretations, it is accepted that what the researcher produces is at least in part a construction, something inherently shaped by the way in which information is collated and themes are represented. It is acknowledged that the researcher cannot but interpret and influence matters (e.g. through the line of questions that they pursue). To illustrate, a researcher exploring perceptions of visits to the dentist first collects the accounts of individuals who have been through this experience. The research interviews have not been rigidly constrained by set questions. Researchers follow lines of enquiry, those that help to clarify their opening ideas gleaned from past interviews. In explaining this (the audit trail), the researcher asks the reader to determine whether the research findings still seem trustworthy and valuable, as they return to the experience in question themselves. This might mean that you, as the reader, think again about what patients tell you, and it might guide some additional questions that you pose to them.

Remember that here, the concern is with the insight and understanding of a phenomenon, not with predicting what will happen in the future. So, the first question you should consider asking is whether or not there is a clear audit trail that describes how data were collected and analysed (Tracey, 2019). Was this by interview or by observation, and in what order? How were the themes reported in the research arrived at? While all researchers need to describe the research design and steps taken, audit trailing is especially important in this paradigm. This is because the researcher presents their own 'take on reality'. Even if the researcher has laid out an adequate audit trail of their work, you might still question whether they have adequately considered all of the possible interpretations of the chosen phenomena. Your test in this regard is whether something that seems important – from your own experience – has been considered. In this paradigm, the researchers believe that the world has potentially infinite experiences, interpretations and perceptions to report. They claim to capture some of these and invite your comparison from personal and professional experience. So, research evidence here might seem incomplete; it might miss something that you believe is important, especially in your practice context. Now the practice utility test is about completeness and fit of research design and evidence to clinical circumstances and needs. You are at liberty to observe, 'Ah, but have you thought about …?' or, 'In this context, patients are usually more concerned about ….' As a reader of this sort of research, you are invited to think again, to focus afresh upon the phenomena in question. I tested this idea out with Raymet, asking her about audit trailing and why this was important in naturalistic paradigm research:

I think it's because researchers here accept that a lot of the important things which nurses are interested in cannot be proven, they cannot easily be measured. After all, being ill is extremely personal. Because of that, the researcher has to access the patient's experiences, which means they have to use a mix of questions, they need to find ways to relate to the patient. So, when I come to judge this research, I want to know about how they did that. I can then say, given my personal experience of illness or patients in the past, this does or doesn't sound convincing.

As Raymet suggests, as well as asking questions about the audit trail, whether or not it was clear how the researchers proceeded, you also need to ask a question about authenticity: 'Given what I already know about this practice, do these findings seem credible?' (Pope and Mays, 2020). Of course, experiences elsewhere might not accord with your personal experience. They might be quite unique to another group of patients or practitioners. But if the research evidence is to be transferable, this concern with authentic, recognisable experience remains important. Quite a lot of naturalistic paradigm research evidence falters at this point. Human experience is contextual; it operates within a particular healthcare system. It may be authentic to local contexts, but it might not be transferable.

Questions in the critical theory paradigm

As critical theory research is polemical, consciously political, the first questions to ask here are: Are the researchers' premises about the need, problem or opportunity set out at the start? What is the research meant to correct or achieve? Honest critical theory paradigm research acknowledges from the outset what has framed and directed the research (Torres and Nyaga, 2021). The critical theory researcher would point out that truth is always contested, that the definition of what is happening is fought over. So, every position is in some sense partial, and reality is defined in terms favourable to the group holding power. However, they concede a responsibility to set out their alternative truth, what they wish to challenge. Having ascertained that the researchers' premises and assumptions are clear, the critical analysis of evidence moves to an audit trail, as above. How was the research conducted? Were the procedures here conducted in accord with the stated purpose of the research and the values of the researchers?

I discussed *action research*, a common method used within critical theory paradigm research, with Gina. She had seen action research under way in a clinic where she had recently been on practice placement. The research was all about developing a more consultative clinic, one that facilitated screening of sexually transmitted infections and contacts that the patient may have had. The researchers had stated that they felt the practitioners there were disempowered, being set targets and standards for the tracing of contacts, but with little help given on how to create an atmosphere more conducive to screening and tracing work. The researchers negotiated a series of activities, first to help the staff examine their concerns and needs, as well as the training that they might require. A second round of activity explored with them their values and attitudes towards risk and patient needs. Patients sought a degree of privacy, but the staff too needed to minimise risk for others, so work centred on facilitating responsibility in the patients. Gina observed:

> *It was egalitarian research; it did attend to staff needs and concerns, but it didn't lose sight of responsibility. Staff did have a duty of care to individual patients and they did have a public health responsibility too. So, in that sense, what the researchers did hold true to their stated values and goals without alienating the managers who had set targets in the first place. It was about how to work better.*

Reviewing critical theory paradigm research, then, is different to that linked to the naturalistic paradigm (which focuses on authenticity of the account) and radically different to that of the positivist paradigm (with its emphasis on reliability and validity). Here, the researcher acknowledges what they consider inequitable, unjust and problematic, as well as describing often collaborative research fieldwork designed to put things right. This has the propensity to make you think about your beliefs and values. Was this endeavour necessary? Do I share the beliefs and concerns of the researcher, and do I believe that their research aids in improving matters? In this paradigm, research does not stand aloof from politics and ideological debates; it drives straight in and provokes questions about the worthiness, the necessity, of particular healthcare.

The nature of evidence-based practice

The discussions above illustrate why research evidence is by no means a simple thing; it comes in many different forms and has been conceived of in different ways. You will need to reason at a high level (see Table 3.1 in Chapter 3) to do justice to a discussion of different sorts of research evidence. The purpose of research may be quite different, depending on how the research was conceived and where the information came from. For example, much research evidence within the naturalistic paradigm has been gathered to facilitate reflection. It raises questions such as 'Have you thought about this?' and 'Does this happen where you work?' Evidence associated with the positivist paradigm may contest current treatment or care; it might suggest what else works better, and the implicit questions are, then, 'Should we do something different?' and 'Should we continue doing this now?'

Evidence associated with the critical theory paradigm relates specifically to attitudes and values, the agendas and beliefs that might shape healthcare. Accepting the complexity of this, the questions posed, suggests that evidence-based practice will not be a one-size-fits-all matter either. Evidence-based practice may consist of changed care because a critical mass of what works, as well as knowledge about what is safe and critical to the improvement of the patient's condition, has accrued.

Evidence from the positivist paradigm is drawn upon, especially where that also accommodates consideration of the costs of healthcare. But evidence-based practice might also involve different ways to conceive of care partnerships, ways of working that show greater sensitivity to the needs of others. Evidence from the naturalistic or critical theory paradigms might be important here. Improvement in nursing care is still the central concern, but it is associated with different things, such as sensitivity, attuning care to patient requirements.

Successful evidence-based practice is, then, that which works with the strengths of different sorts of evidence, provided in association with different paradigms (Linsley and Kane, 2022). There is recognition of the limitations of evidence, as well as what may be claimed about it. Nurses and other practitioners realise that evidence still requires interpretation and decisions about where and how best to use it. Evidence cannot substitute for clinical judgement and critical thinking. They need to be combined with these, and to strategic purpose.

Fundamental challenges usually remain:

- Have we got enough evidence?
- Does it all point in the same direction and suggest broadly the same things?
- Have we got a mix of evidence that attends to the aspects of care, what works, what is safe, and what reassures the patient?
- Is the evidence usable?

Chapter summary

You have now reached the end of Chapter 8 and your exploration of a particular sort of critical thinking, that which applies to evidence and its application in practice. Evidence is one of the key knowledge bases on which nurses draw. It is extremely important and yet hotly contested. If you are to critically examine evidence, it is necessary to understand what sorts of evidence there are, how these are related to paradigms of knowledge, and which questions are appropriate to employ there.

(Continued)

(Continued)

In this chapter, you have explored why both theory and research evidence might have to pass a utility test. Then you have explored different conceptions of evidence. To make sense of sometimes fiercely contested debates on evidence-based practice, you have looked at three paradigms, each of which shapes the ways in which people think about knowledge and conceive of evidence. Asking the right questions of evidence starts with an understanding of paradigms and remains mindful of practice utility, what works in a given clinical context.

Activities: brief outline answers

Activity 8.1   Reflection (page 123)

Post Covid-19 pandemic, in the face of ageing populations, and with growing consumerism in healthcare, questions have arisen about the adequacy or otherwise of care services. Much of that debate itself starts with wildly different assumptions about what a healthcare service should provide. I believe though that it's difficult to think of such service and nursing care as a homogenous whole. I suspect that your clinical placements have already demonstrated that to you. The work of high dependency care, that in the community, that associated with mental health for example, are all very different. It's very difficult to determine what nursing care should be unless we also scrutinise public expectations and priorities. If care is a partnership then we had better understand what the partner hopes for and what they contribute too.

This sets remarkable challenges for healthcare research as well. How realistic is it to design research that produces evidence of a wide application? If, conversely, we accept the importance of context and research is focused upon individual environments, how do we overcome the potential scatter gun effect of evidence? Lots of small studies in individual areas might be difficult to summate let alone action. My argument is then that if evidence-based practice is to be prescriptive, we need to work with widely agreed essential components of most care. Beyond that evidence might prosaically be informative, commending further reflection and offering possibilities for exploration.

Further reading

Aveyard H, Preston, N and Farquhar, M (2023) *How to read and critique research: a guide for nursing and healthcare students.* London: Sage.

No single chapter within a book such as mine can entirely explore research design and methodology, so this is an excellent further study book. It offers advice on critiquing different research designs that are labelled 'qualitative research' as well as those in other paradigms.

Useful websites

http://consumers.cochrane.org

The Cochrane Consumer Network is an offshoot of the original Cochrane Collaboration and is designed to help members of the general public become involved in the evaluation of healthcare evidence. There is excellent guidance on how members of the public can access research evidence, working through the complex terminology there.

www.cochrane.org/about-us

The Cochrane Collaboration provides an extensive collection of systematic reviews of research evidence and a free-to-access handbook on how to plan these. Systematic reviews are rigorous methodological interrogations of intervention research that are usually associated with what effects an intervention has.

Chapter 9   Writing the analytical essay

Chapter aims

After reading this chapter, you will be able to:

- determine clearly the purpose of the analytical essays you write;
- identify the cases presented by others and what you will deliberate upon;
- adopt a clear position on the case within your analytical essay;
- select relevant evidence and link this to arguments within your written work;
- demonstrate more speculative and scholarly ways of writing in your essays;
- prepare conclusions that both sum up previous texts and demonstrate what you deduce from them.

Introduction

Writing essays is a perennial part of learning to nurse, as coursework and in examinations. There is little room for absolute thinking, where you advocate only one cause, where you neglect the options, opinions and debates that encircle nursing practice. You will need to write in a critical way.

This chapter combines my previous teaching on critical thinking and writing, and applies it to analytical essays. I remind you of some of the characteristics of more critical thinking that you first met in Table 3.1 in Chapter 3. I consider the purposes to which the analytical essay is put and highlight the importance of clearly establishing your position before you start writing. I review how best to discriminate what should be included in the essay, and then the use of arguments that demonstrate your ability to weigh the merits and limitations of a case. I revisit how best to sum up the essay within the conclusion, and make the point that success here consists of much more than simply repeating what has been presented earlier in the paper.

The purpose of analytical essays

Analytical essays are set for different purposes. The first of these is to test your understanding of a given subject and your ability to make a series of judgements about it (the evaluative essay). Such essays are frequently set as a review of the literature, research reports or healthcare policies (Fisher et al., 2020). Examiners wish to understand whether you have a clear grasp of what others have argued, and whether you have developed a clear perspective of your own. Evaluative essays are sometimes set early on within a course to check your grasp of key concepts.

The second purpose of the analytical essay is to move forward from this, to assess your strategic thinking: what would you do next, and why (Harrison and McManus, 2017)? A strategic essay might set you a clinical problem or invite you to weigh conflicting demands before advocating your own best course of action. It may test your ability to make choices and the ordering of work in a logical sequence.

The third purpose is to test your ability to confront conundrums or to examine professional ethos (the philosophical essay) (Neff, 2019). Essays of these kind often test your highest-level reasoning skills (see Table 3.1 in Chapter 3) because you have to ruminate on values, attitudes, priorities and principles in a way that shows you are thinking about care as a whole (i.e. in metacognition). Papers about ethical dilemmas may be of this kind.

Activity 9.1   Critical thinking

Below are some essay assignment questions or instructions. Decide which purpose each of these questions serves.

1. The attached case study describes the experiences of Avril, a 35-year-old woman with learning difficulties. She lives within a home with five other residents. Read the account of Avril's relationship with Tony, another resident, and then critically discuss the challenges that arise in association with contraception here.
2. 'Nurses are necessarily interpreters of healthcare policies.' With reference to a policy of your own choosing, critically discuss whether you support this statement. Remember to back up your points with reference to the literature and/or observations from practice.

3. As part of a new initiative to engage the public in strategic healthcare planning, four ex-patients have become consultants to your nursing team. How will you work with them to enhance the services delivered to patients? Make sure that you refer to theories of leadership and change agency taught during your course.

My answers to this activity are given at the end of the chapter.

The case and the position taken

Having established the purpose of the forthcoming essay (what the question asks), our next job is to determine what position we take and what case will be considered (Bailey, 2022). The two are not necessarily the same. A case might be stated as part of the question and you are asked to examine it. Question 2 in Activity 9.1 does just that; the case is stated briefly, simply, that nurses are interpreters of healthcare policies. You present questions and arguments that explain your position on this given case. In other instances, you make the opening case in the essay and back this up with arguments. Under examination conditions, being clear about the case and your position is critical. However, we are often so keen to make the best use of the time available that we set to quickly, writing down points that are confused. Yet we know that by the end of the essay, our position has to be very clear. For example, relating to Activity 9.1, we might decide that we support the statement in question 2 about nurses interpreting policy, but with certain caveats. There are some restrictions because nurses must simultaneously apply several policies and each demands priority attention (what you have learned about assessing information utility in Chapter 8 will be relevant here). You might support the case that nurses interpret policy, but your position is a qualified one. It is vital, then, before you write, even in an examination, to pause and consider what your position will be. If you have the chance to make a case of your own, what will that be?

Activity 9.2   Reflection

Stewart confided in me that he did not always clarify his position before writing essays. He feared that examiners might judge him negatively if his perspective did not mirror theirs. He tried to write an answer that he hoped might please the examiner.

Reflect now on whether this worry has affected you too. Is it as important a problem as not knowing what your position is in the first place? Once you have done this, look back at Table 3.1 in Chapter 3 to remind yourself that in academic settings, the last thing that assessors expect is for you to present an absolute case, one which does not consider other possibilities.

As this answer is based on your own observation, there is no outline answer at the end of the chapter.

Establishing your position is important. This is because it will determine what arguments you make within the essay and what evidence you draw on. Some positions require a great deal of evidence to support them, reflecting the complexity of nursing care. If we continue with the above example, we would need to identify circumstances where:

- we definitely should interpret the chosen policy;
- there is more limited scope to interpret the policy;
- factors combine to severely restrict our ability to interpret the policy.

On balance, if we support the case, the first group of these factors should predominate. Showing that other factors intervene, though, and that there are caveats to consider, demonstrates that our judgement is not rash. In an essay such as this, we might draw on evidence from the literature that is connected to local protocols and standard care pathways, as well as observations from practice and discussions with fellow students who have managed policy implementation in the past.

Activity 9.3   Critical thinking

What sort of brief answer plan might you use in an examination situation to help you prepare an answer that demonstrates your position clearly in response to a question? Jot down an idea or two, perhaps describing a plan that you use now.

My suggested plan is given at the end of the chapter.

Arguments and evidence

We have already seen in Chapter 3 that an essay is composed of a series of sections (introduction, main text, conclusion), which are in turn made up of a sequence of paragraphs, within which we advance our arguments. Coherent essays have arguments that fit with the position being defended and they lead appropriately to the conclusion. Arguments usually include the word 'because', which helps to link the case to the underpinning premises. In essays, however, not every one of your arguments will be constituted that formally. Sometimes you will present opinions or perspectives. Your arguments, though, will still need to be supported by evidence.

We might arrange the essay in several ways; for example, reviewing the alternative positions that might be adopted with regard to nurses' interpretation of healthcare policy, before revealing the position that evidence seems to support. Alternatively, our position may seem so strong that we state this at the outset, and then lead the reader through stepwise arguments that demonstrate its power. A committed stance of this kind is not simply absolute thinking. The case is backed up by a series of carefully considered arguments in support of it. Some evidence is adopted, and other evidence is challenged as being unclear, poorly articulated or perhaps less relevant to the question. The assessor is left in no doubt that you have pondered your answer with care.

It is disempowering to feel that the only arguments which can fairly be advanced in an essay are those that are supported within the literature. This appears to suggest that the only valid form of knowledge is that which has been published. In truth, a significant amount of evidence remains unpublished, and this includes some research findings, audits of practice and observations made in practice. There are different sorts of evidence (Whitman et al., 2017; see also Chapter 8). Before you can couple evidence with your chosen arguments, you need to ascertain how powerful the evidence is and whether it clearly supports the point that you wish to make. A poorly selected piece of evidence can undermine your essay.

Activity 9.4 Critical thinking

Look at the following examples of evidence coupled with arguments that you might include within an essay on interpreting local healthcare policy. Determine whether you think the evidence supports the chosen argument. Then decide whether the pairings seem convincing to you.

1. *The argument:* Nurses are confident enough to examine policies critically because they are acquainted with the legal, ethical and practical constraints that apply to it.

    The evidence: Nurse researchers report in a journal article their grounded theory research, which included interviews with and observations of nurses in practice. The research articulates how nurses action policies.

2. *The argument:* Nurses have advanced some areas of the chosen policy and delayed others, acknowledging that patients are ill-equipped to partner every aspect of care.

    The evidence: A series of audit case studies have been compiled locally that itemise which elements of shared decision-making patients expect to engage in and which they have misgivings about.

3. *The argument:* Nurses have limits set on policy interpretation because older policies are still in place and have not yet been updated to help facilitate the proposed way forward.

    The evidence: Two standard care pathways in operation in local clinical areas are cited as examples of situations where practitioners sometimes express their frustration.

My reflections are given at the end of the chapter.

Deciding which arguments and evidence make it into your essay is critical. You may have previously encountered essay feedback where the tutor has told you that your account was 'too superficial'. You are likely to be guilty of this if you try to include too many arguments and pieces of evidence. The exasperated assessor might observe, 'You seem to record everyone else's position but not arrive at a perspective of your own!'

This is often a problem where you have not shown due regard to the specific circumstances alluded to within the essay question. Remember that higher-order critical reasoning shows greater precision; it is contextualised as well as inquisitive.

Fatima told me about her tendency to set down a large number of fragment arguments, points on the page that didn't show how evidence supported her arguments or else arguments that assume the reader shared common values to herself. Her tutor called this 'mosaic writing', hoping that the reader would make sense of the whole by the end of the essay. Writing fewer but better selected arguments helped her improve grades.

In essays that require you to review a literature (the evidence) it is important that you set out clearly where you looked for relevant material (Wallace and Wray, 2021). Some of your arguments in this essay context will relate to strategy, how many papers were reviewed and why. Within most module-based assessments you aren't required to complete a systematic review of the literature, for example that done within the Cochrane databases, but you nonetheless need to state the limits of your search. Did the review for instance relate to one policy or several pertaining to a group of patients? Did you admit into your review audit material or case studies of policy in action, as well as research reports?

Speculating successfully

Something that students find very difficult to achieve within an essay is speculation. If arguments are founded upon evidence, and evidence is contradictory or even absent, how do we proceed? We are left to rehearse what could be happening or what might be done next. We need to identify what can be suggested, whether that is within the literature or as part of clinical experience. We also need to imagine the future, how services might change, what patient needs could be, and how we might work better with relatives. Speculation is an important part of higher-level critical thinking. Nursing practice needs nurses who are confident and willing to speculate, to imagine what might be the case, what could be required. Failing to ask the right questions often means that opportunities for improvements in practice are lost. In Table 3.1 in Chapter 3, the highest level of critical thinking is demonstrated by asking imaginative questions in care situations.

To speculate with confidence, we need to use terms which signal to the reader that we have moved into speculative mode. If we signal these matters clearly and then write in a measured way about the subject (i.e. without stating what we think is 'obvious' or 'self-evident', or what 'naturally follows'), we will be taking the reader along with us, reasoning at our side.

The following words and short phrases all signal that we are speculating:

- *Notionally*: This suggests that we are considering an embryonic idea – one still in development. For example: 'Notionally, nurses do more to interpret policies than they realise. Even simple care involves interpreting what equals quality.'

- *Arguably*: This is used to suggest that the point is sufficiently clear and coherent to constitute an argument, but it is one we are still considering. For example: 'Nurses' frustration with policy is arguably to do with constraints on professional freedom.'
- *We might speculate*: This is a tentative way of putting things, suggesting an area of enquiry or a line of reasoning. For example: 'We might speculate that while standard care plans save nurses' time, they also limit thinking.'
- *A number of possibilities present*: This sets out possible explanations. For example: 'A number of possibilities present: first, colleagues insist on writing their own policies; second, they form alliances with policymakers; and third, they lament change but persevere with their instructions.'
- *It would be possible to suggest*: This hints that what is written about next has some credibility. For example: 'It would be possible to suggest that nurses are shaping the policies which matter – those that determine the experience of care.'
- *Conceivably*: This suggests something that could be considered but might not be the easiest explanation. For example: 'Conceivably, nurse entrepreneurs are those who see policy as a lever. They use it to achieve desirable ends.'

Activity 9.5   Reflection

Look back over some past essays and note whether you used any of the above words or phrases to indicate that you were speculating. Did you use the words in the right way?

As this answer is based on your own observation, there is no outline answer at the end of the chapter.

Reaching successful conclusions

A large majority of analytical essays written by students describe what has gone before within the essay, but without necessarily demonstrating a conclusion. To use a simple analogy, we describe a journey made (we spent three hours on the train). What is usually required within an analytical essay is to determine the significance of that journey. We can illustrate this by referring to the three purposes of analytical essays described earlier:

- *Evaluative*: The journey was arduous, took longer than expected, and prompted us to reconsider the advantages of using public transport in the future.
- *Strategic*: There remain opportunities to improve upon the journey, at least with regard to the time taken. Weekday public transport schedules are better.
- *Philosophical*: Travelling by public transport had the advantage of reducing our carbon footprint. Had we driven there, the environmental penalty would have been higher.

A successful conclusion, then, must capture the account of what has been written so far (the journey) but must also include a deduction. We have to make clear what matters seem settled and what remain open at the end of the essay. Contrary to what some students think, it is not always true that we need to have 'nailed our colours to the mast', either wholeheartedly adopting or rejecting the case presented to us by others in a question. We do, however, need to have clarified our position: 'The case seems supportable to this extent, but what we need to ascertain further is XYZ.'

In the following example of a concluding paragraph relating to the essay on policy interpretation, there is a clear indication of the author's resting position at the end. Notice how the author refers back to the case that has already been introduced at the start of the essay:

At the start of this paper, I introduced the case that nurses do interpret policies, but cautioned that their success in this is affected by factors that limit their freedom to proceed at will. The paper highlights that pressure of time and the need to serve a public, as well as individual patients, to work effectively in teams and to attend to employer agendas, all shape the interpretation of healthcare policy. My chosen policy (rehabilitation) espouses a philosophy of co-operation and consultation. Nurses might wish to interpret this policy as an opportunity to deliver individualised care, but they do not always have the scope to proceed in that way. Instead, they need to ration their expertise and attention.

In this conclusion, the journey is summed up quickly in the sentence describing what limits nurses' opportunities to interpret policy. The telling point arrives at the end, where it is explained that the nurse might wish to interpret policy in a particular way (as individualised care), but that care is necessarily rationed. The nurse does a little for the many and not as much as might be wished for the few. The author defends the opening case.

Drafting the essay and checking it

Students vary in their preferred ways of writing and editing. Having prepared an outline plan that signals the key sections of the paper, the arguments and evidence that will appear in each, the case that will be considered and the position adopted, some quickly set down a first draft. Students may have checked that they remain within the word counts they have allocated for each section, but they will leave any references, tables and quotes to be added later. The first goal for such students is to get work down on paper that captures their understanding of the subject and which represents their position regarding it. Other students move much more incrementally, carefully crafting each section and adding embellishments as they go. However you proceed, though, checking the clarity and coherence of what has been written remains a responsibility.

I asked the four case study nursing students about their essay drafting and reviewing processes:

Gina: If you write a 'rough' draft of your essay in one sitting, you have the advantage that you don't pause to fret over doubts as you go. Afterwards, though, you need to check whether the arguments stack up.

Fatima: Lately I have worked more with my plan, especially as regards the word allowance. If one section seems tight and I need to include more words than I hoped, I stop right then and ask whether I'm trying to cover too much.

Raymet: I write first draft essays in the morning and then talk the content of my essay through with a friend. I explain what I am arguing. If they seem clear about my thoughts, even if they don't agree with my position, I feel encouraged.

Stewart: Writing for me is private, but I always leave several days to complete an edit. My later essays have been better for that.

I agree with Gina that doubts can creep in as you write. Sometimes work grinds to a halt if you do not write a little more quickly and freely in the first instance. There is something to be said, then, for writing a first complete but more rudimentary draft. It probably captures your position most cleanly, provided that you have allocated enough thinking time before starting work.

Fatima's approach is much more 'sculpted'. The work proceeds in sections and each is 'got right' before the next is attempted. She has moved on from mosaic writing. The approach does produce work that has well-balanced sections, spreading the allocation of words allowed. Students sometimes discover their position shifting a little as they write in this way. It is then necessary to check what is claimed in the introduction – do you still support that?

I especially support Raymet's strategy of summarising a first draft essay. Notice that Raymet sticks to her guns once she has identified what her position will be. This is commendable, provided you have heard and considered the questions and challenges posed by others. Your friend might not have read what you have or attended the lectures that you did, so their position on a subject cannot be yours. Against that, naive questions and thoughtful challenges from reviewers are valuable, as you might well have missed something. To avoid charges of academic collusion and dishonesty, resist the temptation to ask them to edit your essay. This should remain your own work.

If you have left insufficient time to review work, or are preparing several papers in quick succession, essay editing can seem a bit of a chore. It is tempting to submit the work and hope. Time spent checking, however, is beneficial in several ways. You can:

- conduct the spelling, syntax and other presentational checks;
- ensure that the work answers the question or attends to the task set;
- assure yourself that a case has been made – one that is supported, rejected or seen as conditional within the conclusion.

Before closing this chapter, I want to remind you of the importance of representing your sources (citing where they come from) and using quotes in a clear and consistent way. I introduced the risks of plagiarism in Chapter 3, but your last checks on the essay that you have prepared can help you to avoid unwittingly committing plagiarism.

Remember that if in doubt, it is always better to ask a tutor about your work, whether a particular passage avoids plagiarism. Once the work is submitted, you are attesting that what you have provided includes clear attribution of all sources. The most common cases of plagiarism investigated are those associated with inadequate citation and failing to represent the exact words of others accurately using quotation marks (Price, 2014).

Citing others' work

Remember that it is your responsibility to adequately represent where information has come from, irrespective of whether it is published or unpublished, whether it comes from a website or a book/journal, or whether the work is that of your tutor, senior colleagues at work or your employer (Price, 2014). Sources may be primary (where the information is first presented) or secondary (where the original information is summarised by another). It is usually best to represent the original reference where available, by indicating the author(s) name and the year of publication within your text, next to the point that they make. If in doubt, repeat that citation in more than one place – saying that you cited the source three pages ago is not sufficient. If you do use a secondary source, it is important to represent both sources in brackets (author A cited in author B's work, and date). Sometimes students rely quite heavily on a secondary author because they summarise points rather well. You would, though, plagiarise that second author's work if you used their words without clear citation in your text and without the use of quotation marks. Secondary authors' words are not a substitute for your own critique.

As I indicated in Chapter 3, it is necessary to find a balance of others' words and your own reasoning within an essay. A work full of quotes and little analysis of your own will not win you plaudits. Sometimes then it is necessary to paraphrase the work of another author, perhaps because you wish to express their point rather more succinctly, or to quickly connect it to arguments made by other authors. Students sometimes become confused about paraphrasing, the process of summarising others' arguments in your own words. If you use their exact words, this represents a quote, so check that you have enclosed the passage in quotation marks and cited the source, as above. If you have changed their words to your own, then you still need to cite the source. The fact that you have added an interpretation or a new combination of words does not absolve you from that responsibility. Just how many words need to be changed for a paraphrase not to require quotation marks is sometimes debated (Price, 2014). However, I suggest that you create brand new sentences, and that you avoid passages of words which the other author used. Clearly, if they present a key term (e.g. 'person-centred history taking'), that has to be included. But be bold – translate what they say into something that is your own. Here is one last illustration:

> *Original text passage.* Patient anxiety is not only associated with the threat posed (e.g. an operation, a clinical procedure), but with the patient's predisposition

to be fearful. The human brain processes potential threat and potential pleasure within the amygdala. In some instances, life experiences may predispose the individual to anticipate threat more than pleasure.

Adequate paraphrase: Patients are sometimes predisposed to identify threat within a wide variety of situations met. Irrespective of how painful or risky a treatment is (actual threat), they can still be fearful (surname of original author and date).

Once you have completed the last citation and quotation requirements, check that all your references appear in the list at the end of your work, and that the details included in the text (surname and date) match that which is included in your reference list.

Chapter summary

Each individual essay is a work that operates in context, attending to the question or task set. Even though this is an academic work, it still expresses your preferred ways of working. You are the person who drafts the work and you write in a way that enables you to present scripts on time. There are, however, certain features of good analytical essay writing that show your critical thinking at work. You need to be very clear about the purpose of the essay and to write in the appropriate way. Are you going to evaluate or philosophise, for example? You need to determine what case is being discussed and what position you take on it. In some instances, an examiner will set the case by making an assertion that you are invited to evaluate. In other instances, you select a case of your own – one that you will defend using arguments and evidence as your essay unfolds. Good analytical essay writing includes sufficient arguments and pieces of evidence to make a clear case. There is a balance struck between analytical writing (what you think) and descriptive writing (what you report). Where the debate remains open and the best way forward is still to be discovered, you will make selective use of more speculative forms of writing. Conclusions are arranged in such a way that they do more than describe what has been discussed in the text. They indicate where your reasoning has led. All of this is improved where you allocate sufficient time to editing your own work.

Activities: brief outline answers

Activity 9.1   Critical thinking (page 136)

1. This is a tricky one. There are ethical and philosophical issues at stake here surrounding human and reproductive rights, so the essay has a philosophical purpose. It is strategic too, though, as challenges in this instance seem to pose the question 'What will you do next?' In these instances, the clues to what may be required often exist in the case study.

2. The purpose here is evaluative. The opening assertion, about nurses interpreting policy, makes this clear. Do you support this case?

3. The purpose here is strategic. The essay requires you to write about how you might involve lay consultants in the business of care delivery.

Activity 9.3   Critical thinking (page 138)

One plan that I have found workable is as follows:

- Essay purpose: what is asked of me?
- Case made: mine or the examiner's (name it)?
- My position: for or against the case, caveats noted.
- Section 1: introduction and signposting.
- Section 2: main body.
- Key arguments and paired evidence (argument 1, evidence; argument 2, evidence; etc.).
- Section 3: conclusions.

Activity 9.4   Critical thinking (page 139)

Did you notice how some of the arguments were formally worded, including the word 'because'?

The first argument is really about the potential of nurses to interpret policies because of what they consider as part of that process. The research evidence (grounded theory) illustrates how nurses do this. Whether nurses within your chosen context exhibit the same potential may be debatable.

The second argument is about nurses' judgement. The claim is that policy is implemented to a degree, sometimes because patients are not ready to collaborate in care. In this instance, there is a very good fit of evidence – a local audit has determined what patients feel able to do. The argument is supported if the discussion is about a policy interpreted locally.

The third argument is about constraints. Not all policies are written so as to advance care together. Older policies (in this instance, standard care pathways) are working at odds with the new policy. Once again, the evidence seems a promising match, although it is not inconceivable that nurses might not find an adequate compromise between the old and new policies, and this could represent interpretation of policy.

Further reading

Greetham, B (2022) *How to write better essays (Bloomsbury Study Skills)*, 5th edition. London: Bloomsbury Academic.

Bryan Greetham offers a methodical explanation of the ordering of ideas on the page, and one that complements the chapter you have just read. It's not written specifically for healthcare students, but the explanations hold good.

Wallace, M and Wray, A (2021) *Critical reading and writing for postgraduates*, (Student Success) 4th edition. London: Sage.

While this book is firmly aimed at postgraduate students, a wide range of learners should still find it of value. Both undergraduate and postgraduate students are often asked to 'critically evaluate the literature', weighing up what the balance of literature offers as well as evaluating what individual authors claim. So this can be a dip-into book or a cover-to-cover read as you grow more confident.

Useful website

https://en.wikibooks.org/wiki/Writing_Better_University_Essays

This free-to-access e-book provides a good array of guidance on essay writing in coursework and examination contexts. Although not specifically aimed at healthcare students, the guidance usually holds good as regards the principles of analytical writing. I liked the summary of common problems met with in essay writing.

Chapter 10 Writing the reflective essay

Chapter aims

After reading this chapter, you will be able to:

- identify the important tasks to be attended to when writing a reflective essay;
- explain clearly the purpose of reflective essays;
- demonstrate insights into the reporting of events, feelings, perceptions, perspectives, interpretations, conclusions, and planned next actions associated with reflection;
- critically evaluate the merit of writing using a simple reflective practice framework.

Introduction

As you approach the preparation of a reflective practice essay it's good to remember three things:

- You are reflecting on action rather than reflecting in action (see Chapter 2). For the purposes of your essay the reflection should now be complete and you should have determined a number of things about the episode concerned. If you are reflecting as you write, then quite probably you have not completed the necessary thinking work required.
- The reflective essay is concerned with demonstrating the ways in which you have realised something from practice. If other essays are about demonstrating your command of theory, this essay needs to signal your discoveries (Zafeer et al., 2023). A good reflective practice essay demonstrates how you have begun to theorise, to create explanations of that encountered.
- Whichever reflective framework you use, filling in responses to the various sections of that will not necessarily demonstrate your reflective abilities (see Table 3.2). You will need to show you have brought together your experiences and observations, together with any relevant reading. Even in a reflective practice essay there is room for the inclusion of references from the literature, carefully selected to augment your discoveries.

In this chapter I want to illustrate for you the reasoning process that you might use when preparing your reflective practice essay. I will be using my own chosen reflective framework, that proposed by Rolfe et al. (2011). The three questions, 'what', 'so what' and 'what next?' can be used to create logical sections within your paper. If you are using another framework then it might be appropriate to allocate the first sections of your paper to showing how you have answered the questions posed there. Thereafter a 'discussion' section might be used to link the reflection to wider reading. All reflective essays, however, benefit from a short introduction which helps to set the chosen reflective episode in context. To help with this illustration I have asked two case study students, Gina and Raymet to reflect upon the process with me.

Before you write

Before you reach the essay composition stage there are a couple of things you should have prepared. First you must have identified an episode with describable parameters, that which forms a reflective whole, open to analysis. Usually that means a relatively short episode, albeit perhaps with some preliminary contextual information about what led up to it. So my example centres on completing a patient history with a patient. The episode took less than an hour. An episode that stretched over days or weeks might be much harder to analyse. The second thing that you should ensure is that the episode is open to reflection upon what you thought and did as well as what the patient, relative and or other colleagues did. You cannot stand aloof from the reflective process; this is about you as well as them. Thirdly, it is important to set aside enough think time to reach a position on that reflection, for example, did it represent a success, did it highlight a problem, did the reflection represent a discovery, requiring you to shift perspective in some way? It won't be enough to write the essay and not deduce something from the experience.

Table 10.1 summarises some of the other key considerations as you plan your reflective practice assignment.

Requirement	Notes
Represent enquiry	Your writing will need to sound inquisitive. You should avoid sounding complacent, as though the episode simply confirmed what you already knew. So choose an episode that made you think again, which challenged your assumptions.
Examine facts, perspectives, perceptions, narratives and discourses	You will probably write about all of these but will need to be careful about how you deploy your words. In my working example below, it was a fact that the woman divulged more in interview than I anticipated. Perspectives tend to refer to beliefs, attitudes and values and they are rarely universal, so don't assume all think as you do (Aleshire et al., 2019; Skela-Savič et al., 2017). Perceptions refer to your impressions and they might change over the episode and beyond. Narratives are the way in which we (and others) story the episode, what we think was going on. A discourse refers to something bigger, that which links the episode to major issues (e.g. Secunda et al., 2020), in this instance the discourse is about the right purpose of patient history taking.
Demonstrate insight	You will need to demonstrate how you have been attentive towards others and gained something from any interaction. Empathy, for example, is important in reflective practice writing (Jack and Levett-Jones, 2022).
Respect others	You will need to protect the identity of participants (adjust names) within the episode reviewed and secure their permission to write about the episode. Such assurances are however subject to the requirements linked to protecting the vulnerable and reporting abuse (Hamm, 2021).
Demonstrate learning	Your reflection should look forward to future practice: whatever your chosen reflective framework, there should be a 'so what?' element.

Table 10.1   Reflective Practice essay requirements

Activity 10.1   Reflection

Pause now to think about reflective practice essays that you may have written to date. Did you really decide what you learned, before you started to write? Gina admits that she was often in a hurry to set points down. It was as if her grasp of the episode might slip away if she didn't begin. She decided though that this usually made the essay harder, not easier to write.

As this is a personal reflection activity, no suggested answers are included at the end of the chapter.

Writing the introduction

The purpose of the introduction is to set the scene, to indicate what the text will explore and to persuade the reader that you have something significant to relate. Unlike in the papers discussed within Chapter 9, it is not the role of the introduction to state your case. Instead you will lead the reader to your case at the end of the paper. This is an incremental process, one where you gradually reveal your insights. You might reasonably call this the revelatory approach and it is one that Raymet particularly values as it is in line with her past scholarly writing tradition. You could signal the significance of the paper in several different ways, but I recommend outlining how you have thought afresh about the wisdom of practice in a given subject area. We set out what is often considered normal and then incrementally through the reflective practice sections reveal that things are not as straightforward as they seem.

The episode that I am writing about in my example concerned a patient-history-taking interview completed with a 67-year-old woman called Grace who had suffered a heart attack. She had been stabilised within casualty and then came to the ward for onward assessment and review of different treatment options. Grace is married to Roy, and he waits outside the ward while the history-taking interview takes place. Grace has received treatment for her chest pain and is comfortable enough to talk about the frightening episode. What proves interesting is that Grace not only answers my standard questions about her lifestyle and symptoms but that she launches upon a confession about the months she has spent lying to her husband about her angina. What makes the episode interesting, too, is that her detailed account of her subterfuge is designed to counter Roy's habitual hypochondria and anxiety. The question arises what next? Is the interview any longer simply an information gathering exercise?

Activity 10.2   Critical thinking

Raymet suggested that a good way to introduce this essay would be to highlight that many care interactions are poorly captured by the forms that we fill in. We cannot simply rely on questions that the form directs. What do you think are strengths and the limits of Raymet's suggestion? Jot some points down before reading on.

As this is based on your own reflection, no outline answer is given at the end of this chapter.

I told Raymet that her suggestion was an excellent start. However, as the module of study focused on person-centred care it seemed possible to open with something even stronger than that. What Grace had shared with me went beyond 'form filling'; it raised questions too about the start of the care relationship. Was I, for instance, to collude with her as she sought to manage the heart attack narrative with her husband. So here is what I wrote in the opening paragraph. See whether you think that this makes a promising start against the requirements set out in Table 10.1.

The patient-history-taking interview is important. It serves an obvious information gathering function, securing details that might be important for medical diagnosis and treatment. It is typically one of the first encounters at the start of a new care relationship. Rapport within the care relationship might blossom from a good beginning here. Patient history interviewing though is also important as regards managing care workloads. The patient starts to receive a service and the nurse's enquiries form part of that. We might speculate about how best to deliver service to individual patients while being equitable to others as well. The patient-history-taking interview represents one to one 'quality time' spent with the patient.

Do you see here how I am creating a tension? The patient-history-taking interview should be many different things, but that could become complicated. If I have started well here, then the reader wonders, so what happened next? How did this interview inform these traditional assumptions?

Writing the 'what?'

In my example reflective practice essay the next section is entitled 'what?' Whichever reflective framework you use there needs to be a section that factually and accurately summarises the episode as it unfolded. This needs to be summarised as the assignment word limit won't allow for long passages of 'he said, she said'. You can report what you speculated about at the time, that which shaped your responses, but it is vital to keep this section as factual as possible. It is this material that the reader will use to make sense of your retrospective interpretation (so what?) and why you shaped 'what next' in the way that you did.

I showed Gina some bullet points that I had set out to help me plan this section of the paper. The bullet points covered the opening story that I have shared above, but importantly it also set out the sequence of the interaction. What comes first, what follows afterwards is important in an episode interaction. This is because care is created in real time, as a negotiation and often as here, as a departure from standard practice. What started as a routine information-gathering exercise became an urgent consultation on how Grace preferred to manage information about her illness. It was key to distil the interaction within my bullet points because the 'what?' section of my paper was the most descriptive and I didn't want it to occupy more than 25 per cent of the word allowance. Here are the bullet points:

- Short summary of Grace and her admission via casualty with a confirmed heart attack (coronary artery occlusion). Roy accompanies her but is not present at interview.
- I introduced myself, check on her current level of pain and anxiety and then explained that I needed to gather some details. I couch this exercise as gathering information that might be used to allay her anxieties over the coming days (*my practice template here starts with the premise that if we locate history taking as something that helps reduce anxiety, then we will start well. I assume at outset that she is anxious about herself*).

- I start with some standard questions but when I ask about her marital status she becomes agitated and asks urgently that I help her manage her anxious husband. He always 'sees the worst'. Grace embarks upon a long explanation of angina pain that she has hidden from her husband.
- I divert from my standard questions and ask about her own assessment of the seriousness of her symptoms. But Grace dismisses such concerns and returns to her husband and his worries.
- I ask her then about how she would like us to support Roy and manage information. There will be tests and stents may be fitted very quickly. I am not sure that it is easy to conceal the seriousness of the illness.
- She asks that we relate all information to her and that she will 'translate' that for Roy. (*This felt like an invitation to collude with her.*)
- I suggest that we might discuss an information strategy for Roy a little later on. Right now I am gathering essential information for the treatment to come.
- She insists that she must interpret everything for Roy because he is so anxious. She would prefer that he is asked to go home until the preliminary treatment is finished. I have not committed to follow her requirement as regards communicating with Roy and feel the need to consult.
- Because she grew more tired, I curtailed the interview at that point, but she insists that I must manage Roy her way.

I used the bullet points to write up this second section in paragraph form. In this section there is unlikely to be many references added unless they materially shape how the events progressed.

Activity 10.3   Critical thinking

What are the advantages of planning the 'What?' information in bullet point form? Does this address any of your concerns about summarising the episode?

I offer brief answers at the end of the chapter.

Writing the 'so what?'

It is useful to think of the 'so what?' section of your paper as being about issues: why the episode is significant, interesting or problematic. It's in this section that any lack of essay planning shows most clearly. If you have not distilled in your mind what the episode represents, then muddled thinking will be more noticeable here. So I asked Raymet and Gina to identify what they thought the key issues were and I must say that they captured them well. Here they are (see if you agree):

- There's a question about whether the medical purpose of patient history taking, and the care relationship development purpose collide. What should the interview concentrate upon and is it right to diverge from that?

- There's an understanding of Grace's husband care narrative issue (do we really understand that?) and whether such a narrative is realistic? It seems very unlikely that we can resist Roy's questions about his wife's situation, nor will treatment seem other than major.
- It is possible that Grace was still in shock during the interview, but does she really appreciate the seriousness of her circumstance? Gathering information leads to consultation and that might include alerting colleagues about Grace's insight difficulties.
- This was an interview that might have been extended, to help build rapport with Grace and perhaps to explore the feasibility of her preferred communication strategy. But would that have been timely and equitable to others who also need the nurse's attention?
- Grace's demands could seem like a trap, an insistence upon one strategy, but what does that mean for the 'negotiation of care' in person-centred care? Must we sometimes say no, that is unwise?

Activity 10.4   Investigation

Explore one of the short film patient stories that you will find at www.patientstories.org. uk. Study your chosen film in order to jot down a series of issues that you think arise, that which might involve further thought on what nurses can or should do to help. This is a really good exercise to do as it will practise your in-issue analysis. Nurses need to 'read' the significance of what patients say as well as what a care interaction might tell us. Much of my own chosen reflective practice episode centres upon what Grace said. If possible, compare your issues list with a colleague who also watched the film.

As this is a personal investigation, no outline answer is given at the end of the chapter.

At best your list of issues can become a plan for the paragraphs that will make up the 'so what?' section of your essay. Of course you might have to consider trimming these, focusing on the most important issues if your reflective episode prompted a much longer list. Five issues though (in my example) seemed a realistic array of material to cover within this section of the essay. Each could represent one or two substantial paragraphs, picking out the significance of what I encountered and thought about resulting from the episode.

Gina asked, 'how speculative should you be when you write this section?' This seems a good question. On the one hand you need to signal to the reader that you are not foreclosing on what might be important within the episode. It's likely that your information isn't entirely complete so there are gaps to ponder. I hadn't interviewed Roy, for example, to assess his concerns and needs. Against that though, this has to be a finished piece of writing and the discussion has to be coherent and complete enough to indicate that you have decided what really matters. So here is a short passage of my writing that hopefully illustrates that balance. I am writing about what above was described as Grace's trap.

What impressed about Grace's account of her lies to Roy regarding developing angina and her demands about how we should communicate with him, was what seemed like a well-developed but rigid narrative of coping. This was how she coped with an illness threat, and a partner responsibility, and she was resolute that the coping approach should be reinforced now. The sudden admission to hospital challenged that and the need now for cardiac treatment seemed to threaten her preferred way of doing things. It was certainly the case that I felt trapped, required to respond in Grace's preferred communication. But then again, I had insufficient evidence at this stage to be sure that she would stick with her demands as treatment requirements became clear. It was possible that Grace made her demands while still in a state of shock.

Do you see here how I counterbalance an analysis of what Grace was doing (coping her way) with a doubt about how tenable that was? Care is like this, we move forward with some insights that seem pretty certain, but they might not be absolute and forever. We hadn't as yet recounted what treatment might entail and what longer term adjustments to her life might be wise. Whatever Grace's opening gambit on this negotiation was, she might have to face some questions about what was viable longer term.

Remember this is a section where you might add references from the literature. In this case that might refer to different patterns of patient coping or emotional reaction to a cardiac event (for example, Kroemeke 2016; Peltzer et al., 2022). However, I suggest that you use such references in passing, as indication that you know of research or theory that guides your analysis. If you divert at length to the theory or research your reflective practice essay starts to slip away into literature review.

Writing the 'what next?'

We move now then to 'what next?' and here I think there are two challenges. The first concerns what range and volume of response to the issues are you meant to cover? You could write at length about what the health team do or concentrate on the nursing response. The second challenge relates how prescriptive you are meant to sound, responding to the issues identified. If you are extremely prescriptive, then you might demonstrate the sort of absolutist reasoning that was described as low-level critical thinking in Chapter 3.

My own approach to these challenges is to remind myself (and perhaps the reader) that responses in healthcare often need to be responsive and collaborative. As healthcare is ideally not a standard package prescription (remember that this module centres on person-centred care), so our support and solutions to problems might change over time as all parties reevaluate the care journey together (Price, 2022). So I would concentrate my 'what next?' responses to the period while Grace's health is stabilised. During this period we can realistically hope to help Grace review what has happened and what that means for coping.

I invited Raymet and Gina to suggest what they might commend as regards 'what next?' I reminded them that this might not mean action, treatment and prescription, but might include further enquiry. Nursing care is not like medical prescription where a pathology is completely defined and treatment directed. Instead we explore changing experiences and needs. Happily this can sometimes help us avoid conflict, an either/or impasse.

Gina was in favour of confronting Grace with how unrealistic her preferred coping was. It had increased risk of serious injury to her heart and even death. It was a strategy that longer term wasn't viable as regards a partner. Raymet though argued that rehearsal was a better way to see this matter. What if we helped Grace to rehearse the merits of different coping strategies? I supported Raymet's suggestion, but recommended that we enlist the physician to help with some realistic information sharing to Grace about the incidence and significance of later cardiac episodes. I thought that Grace needed to be appraised honestly of future risk and it was against that we could help her deliberate more accurately on how to cope, with both illness and her spouse.

In the 'What Next?' section then we will need to write about how we respond to the issues raised in the last section. It doesn't always mean prescription, it could mean further enquiry or a new sort of collaboration. Instead of confronting what we believe to be 'the problem' we might reframe it so that Grace can manage it differently. Writing in these ways, in this section, you have a chance to persuade the reader of several important nursing values, those relating to empathy, to compassion and collaboration.

I think it's important to address all the issues that you raise in the preceding section. If you leave some out, and don't explain the need to prioritise, the examiner might easily observe that you have left business unfinished. In this section (as the last) there is scope to draw in some references, some points made from the literature. There is in this instance a fairly rich literature on cardiac rehabilitation and the psychological adjustments that are best made after cardiac episodes (e.g. Nagel et al., 2021). As before though, the literature is used to acknowledge a caution or commend a response. There isn't space within your reflective practice essay to divert for any length of time to discuss research or theory from elsewhere. As Gina put it, 'you have to press literature's nose to the grindstone of the problem'. If you don't do that, you are slipping away from the analysis of practice and what it can teach you.

Activity 10.5   Reflection

Think back now to any reflective practice essays that you have written so far and had marked. Did your work reach a 'what next?' stage and was that something commended in your written feedback? If it was critiqued, have you noticed any trends in the commentary. For example, do you try to cover too many points, leaving each underdeveloped? Are your suggestions for 'what next?' too trite, perhaps idealistic rather than practical? Seeing an assignment as more than a discrete response to one essay is a good way of improving your writing.

As this is a personal reflection, no sample answer notes appear at the end of the chapter.

Writing a conclusion

In some reflective essays set, a conclusion is not required. Instead, the 'what next?' section is designed to demonstrate what you think is concluded and mandated, linked to the episode concerned. A practised senior student can manage that reasonably easily. I think though that for most students, with most earlier stage course assessments, that a conclusion section to the essay is worthwhile. This is because it enables you to overtly link the discoveries made back to the assumed or past practice that you used to introduce the reflection in the first place. Be sure then to check out what the assignment guide requires of you. Do you have to utilise a particular reflective practice framework and are you required to include a conclusion section. Check the word allowance in particular and any remarks made about word allocations to different sections of the essay.

Let us assume that you're writing a conclusion. What are the requirements? Here is what I think:

- You should add no new material into the essay at this stage, but should draw the sections of your paper together.
- It should capture the case that you make, if 'what next?' doesn't exemplify that.
- It should be more than one decent length paragraph and no more than three. That sounds pedantic, but really short conclusions rarely demonstrate your learning, while very long ones suggest that you haven't finished reasoning in the preceding sections. You should have reached a calm and quiet resting place here.

In my example essay I would write a conclusion that stated that while the patient-history-taking interview fulfilled multiple different roles, some of these could come into conflict. The need to gather information and to establish a respectful rapport with the patient does not always work in synchrony. There are 'wild card' elements that can emerge from any care dialogue, but especially an opening one such as this. It is unwise to imagine that we can completely contain the negotiations that might commence during a patient-history-taking interview, but not automatic that we must resolve them there and then. You might have noticed that I concluded the interview without assuring Grace that we would communicate with Roy in precisely her required way.

Notice how that sort of conclusion differs from the standard descriptive one that simply summarises what the essay sections have covered. It has become a substantive conclusion, one which incidentally hints at a revised practice template that I am working towards. That template concerns the opening of care relationships and the need to gather information for stakeholders. We will need to gather useful information, to ascertain the patient's concerns, but it may be unwise to make instant promises.

Chapter summary

In this chapter, I have illustrated for you how one reflective practice framework can help you to shape a clear and coherent reflective practice essay answer. Different frameworks might shape how you create sections within your essay, but what remains key throughout is that you reach some important conclusions about what the episode represented before you start to write. You are reflecting on action and once removed, when there has been time to ponder what happened and what any complementary literature might add.

As in other essays, you will need to make a case, but as this is an essay sharing discoveries, that case typically appears at the end of the essay. The reflective practice essay involves meeting a number of requirements, those relating to enquiry, insight and respect for others for example. However, a successful essay can be produced, one that teaches us that practice can facilitate our reasoning abilities, those associated with speculation and next step future planning as well as reflective scrutiny regarding what has since passed.

Activities: brief outline answers

Activity 10.3   Critical thinking (Page 152)

The chief benefit in using bullet points in this context is that you set the episode in event order, what happened, first, second, third, etc. An episode operates in several different dimensions at once, changing over time (forwards) as we react to what others say and do, and in terms of perceptions of what we think is being negotiated or collaborated upon (discourse). The episode operates in a third direction and that relates to what we do or say and what we think. Because the nurse is right there reflecting in action (real-time reasoning) it is especially important to catalogue the sequence of events as they unfold. Our understanding of others' narratives (and by implication their needs), changes over time. But to appreciate that fully we need to understand why we acted or spoke as we did. Imagine episodes that involve conflict: the discord didn't happen instantly. Classically it happens in a sequence and a context.

When I have tutored students on reflective practice, the use of bullet pointing has often been key to improving their essay work. Writing down bullet points slows down the reflective reasoning, it forces a pause and think moment. I hope that you find bullet pointing equally beneficial.

Further reading

Bassot, B (2020) *The reflective journal*, 3rd edition. London, Bloomsbury Academic.

This volume alludes to different reflective practice frameworks which is useful, but, better still, it majors on the exploration of attitudes, values and beliefs, intimate areas of reasoning for every nurse. The text isn't aimed specifically at nurses, but it is very accessible.

Bolton, G and Delderfield, R (2018) *Reflective practice: writing and professional development*, 5th edition. London: Sage.

Reflective practice and writing are not limited to healthcare, so dipping into this book, which deals with the process more generally, is very valuable. The explanations of perspective and narrative are especially good.

Esterhuizen, P (2023) *Reflective practice in nursing*, 5th edition. London: SAGE/Learning Matters.

This is a good source of information on reflective practice models and the process of reflecting in a methodical way. The text is accessible, practical and reassuringly 'how to'.

Useful website

www.patientstories.org.uk

There is an activity associated with this website earlier in the chapter, but I think it's well worth returning there for a wider understanding of how people experience both illness and care. We operate within a world of healthcare consumerism, where patients are much more active and sometimes vociferous participants in care and treatment negotiations. Taking some time to review and identify some recurring traits in public expectations of healthcare is time well spent, both to understand what we mean by 'need' and to understand why care delivery can sometimes seem so stressful. As you watch the films available here it's worth pondering to what extent the aspirations of patients and nursing coalesce. While reflective practice exists to improve care, and to help you articulate your learning on a course, it exists as well to help you make sense of what practice demands. The better you understand that, the more resilient you may become over a lifetime career in caring.

Chapter 11 Writing the clinical case study

NMC Future Nurse: Standards of Proficiency for Registered Nurses

Because the subject matter of clinical case studies varies so widely, this approach may address almost any of the standards of proficiency for registered nurses. The skills covered in this chapter underpin how you review and build practice templates, ways to approach care in a strategic and ethical manner.

Chapter aims

After reading this chapter, you will be able to:

- explain what a clinical case is, something that captures a patient in a care context;
- summarise what is important when choosing a clinical case to write about;
- set the scene for the clinical case study, capturing the reader's interest in what you have to share;
- explain why the case needs to be explained in a measured and dispassionate way before moving on to analysis;
- outline the role of evidence in the clinical case study;
- characterise the analytical writing needed as you discuss case insights and concerns;
- outline what is required when you write up your conclusions to the clinical case study.

Introduction

In Chapter 6, I highlighted the advantage of following one or more clinical case studies during practice placements on your course. Sometimes the narrative of care that we need to understand extends beyond the single reflective interlude. Sometimes understanding the patient, the evolving care relationship, is more important than understanding the event, especially if you work towards more person-centred care (Price, 2022). Case studies can demonstrate our profound respect for the dignity of the patient, their coping endeavours, sometimes in the face of overwhelming threat or change. Dealing with illness, and supporting patients sometimes represents a marathon, rather than a sprint. Now we come to the writing up of those case studies and some points about the value of the same with regard to critical thinking.

Clinical case studies have remained a recurring feature of medical practice writing, where they have a very clear purpose (see the further reading section at the end of the chapter). The clinical case study is used to spotlight some unusual features of an illness or its management that the author believes will be of professional interest to colleagues (Dickey and Botzer, 2021). The purpose of the clinical case study (sometimes called a report) is to use practice experience to better inform the practice of others. A clinical case study in the medical sense is noteworthy not necessarily because the treatment was successful. Rather, it exists to shed light on what experience, as well as the use of related evidence, can teach us (Honeycutt and Miller, 2021). In the context of this book, clinical case studies have a very useful function, which is to illuminate practice template thinking, the way in which one practitioner (or team) tackled a particular need or problem. Nurses relate to patients as people, negotiating care through perceived needs. That which the patient achieves during care is as much to do with how patients feel and relate to healthcare staff as the efficacy of particular treatment. The nurse negotiates rather than prescribes care. In this, the nursing clinical case study is unique; it centres upon the patient and their context as much as upon an illness and any treatment.

In the past, 'nursing care studies' were written by students, often to illustrate a model of nursing in action. One of the problems of such studies, however, was that they could become unduly descriptive. It was relatively easy to write a simple account of care when what was really required was an illustration of critical thinking. For case study writing to work well, there needs to be a problem analysed, a conundrum explained, an insight gained and reviewed, something that sets the case in context and enables the nurse to demonstrate what is now understood about delivering patient care over a period of time.

Today, a clinical case study can (Price, 2017):

- explore the nature of person-centred care;
- illustrate how experience contributes to best practice;
- examine the linkage of evidence and practice (e.g. the case study might illustrate gaps in evidence or indicate where evidence of different sorts might usefully be combined);
- demonstrate higher-level critical thinking and reflection in action (case studies are an excellent way to explore the practice templates that nurses use to reason care).

Selecting the case

I have already indicated some of the key features of a patient's circumstances that might make them a good case to explore as part of your practice placement learning (see Chapter 6). All of those still hold good, but the selection of which case study to write up for assessment, or perhaps a paper for publication, requires some further thought. Most obviously, the patient's case has to fit with the objectives of a module of study (or else the requirements of a journal). If the module of study is on mental health, then clearly that must feature strongly within the case that you write up. Beyond that, though, there should be something about the case that allows you to demonstrate how you are interrogating experience, exploring the concepts in use and evaluating necessary skills. It is not enough that the patient evoked compassion, that they were articulate or friendly. Study of the patient's circumstances and nursing response has to exhibit how you and other nurses thought differently.

Case study: Elijah, part 1

To explain the planning and writing work with a case study, I am going to share a story about Elijah. Picture a 71-year-old man who suffered from Covid-19 pneumonia, necessitating a two-week stay in an intensive care unit (ICU). Elijah was extremely ill, nursed on a ventilator; and after being weaned off that, he was cared for within a rehabilitation unit, which forms the location for the case study.

In some regards, Elijah had much in common with other Covid-19 victims. The illness exhausted him, and it took a long time for him to improve his lung function afterwards. What was important, however, were some rapidly developing delusions that followed his intensive care experience. Elijah believed that he had been persecuted in the ICU. This centred upon a physiotherapist who was trying to help him recover now. Elijah's rehabilitation was adversely affected by the delirium, and the nature of his heartfelt beliefs that followed his time on a ventilator.

Elijah's case above highlights the importance of finding the right focus for analysis. He has been chosen because his case highlights some problems met during rehabilitation. While there is an established history of delirium associated with ventilator treatment, Elijah's context is more interesting still. Elijah's delirium centred upon some heartfelt fears and beliefs that could damage his chances of a successful rehabilitation. In his case, the delirium did not present as a general agitation, sometimes described as 'hyperactive delirium' (Ala-Kokko et al., 2022); it focused firmly upon his delusions. Elijah's rehabilitation relied upon breathing exercises but those could not progress well until his concerns were adequately investigated, delusions and delirium explained, and trust rebuilt.

Activity 11.2   Reflection

Classically, the case chosen centres on an unusual patient circumstance or care response. The patient's story highlights the unusual, perhaps as regards need or care solution. But there is no reason why a case study might not become the vehicle for something even nearer to home, the challenges of sustaining nursing care in the face of significant adversity. Elijah's story, and the nature, extent, of the nursing response could be used to examine the limits of nurse resilience under exacting circumstances. Jot down what you think that a Covid-19 pandemic case such as Elijah's might illuminate as regards nurse resilience.

I offer my speculations at the end of the chapter.

Writing the context introduction

University requirements for the setting out of clinical case studies may vary, but I would recommend an introduction that sets the context of the case study. The role of the introduction is to bring to the reader's attention why this case study is noteworthy. What about the patient or their care marks the work as remarkable in some regard? Classically, case studies are introduced for the following reasons:

- they highlight a previously poorly articulated or unmet problem that deserves analysis;
- they exemplify a feature of care negotiation, perhaps that which illuminates care philosophy or a key skill;
- they highlight something important about the interface between evidence and practice, or perhaps between theory and that which is realisable in care;
- they articulate the resolution of dilemmas.

While clinical case study writing should be measured and analytical, this does not mean that it should be introduced drily. The introduction should interest the reader. The case study may be an assignment answer, but it should have professional merit too – it should seem valuable to another nurse.

In the example of Elijah, several contexts seem important. The first concerns delirium and recovery after time spent on a ventilator. Delirium takes different forms; it may be hyperactive (classically, the patient is agitated and anxious), or hypoactive (the patient is withdrawn and difficult to engage with) (Dubiel et al., 2022). But to varying degrees, too, the patient might experience hallucinations and delusions about what happened in the ICU or what is happening now. The question arises: how shall we best counter delirium?

The second context relates to care philosophy. Like other Covid-19 victims, Elijah faced an acute admission to hospital that quickly deteriorated into an emergency situation where he required mechanical ventilation. There was scant time for nurses to build a rapport with Elijah, to negotiate care in an adequately person-centred way. Care negotiation had to play catch-up after a frightening experience. The question arises: how do you make care person-centred in these circumstances?

The third context was associated with Elijah's background. As a man of colour, as well as being at risk from Covid-19 because of his age and gender, Elijah faced considerable uncertainty. It was important, then, to support him in a sensitive way, reassuring him as much as possible. He experienced ICU care as a racially linked threat. Helping Elijah had to involve understanding his perceptions of events and appreciating the cultural sensitivities that this might involve.

Here is an extract paragraph from the introduction to the case study where I try to capture the reader's professional interest in this case.

Case study: Elijah, part 2

Nurses hope to partner patients in care, to negotiate care measures from a position of mutual respect. Sometimes, however, person-centred care relationships must start from another place, one where it is exceptionally hard to empower patients. Sometimes the care negotiations begin where the patient feels disempowered, suspicious, and where the nurse must use all of their skills to help the patient feel secure. Whatever best practice guidelines we have for person-centred care, they presume a collaborative starting point. When a 71-year-old patient, Elijah (name adjusted), is admitted to hospital acutely ill with Covid-19-related pneumonia, however, where they are rapidly transferred to the ICU and artificial ventilation, the care negotiating begins post-traumatic event. Care is negotiated against a significant power imbalance where the patient is severely disadvantaged. It is then heightened further when efforts to build rapport with the patient during rehabilitation are complicated by delirium, the patient rapidly developing a series of delusions about his ICU care and the motives of a therapist who is trying to assist him with his breathing and mobility exercises now.

Activity 11.3   Critical thinking

Compare the above opening paragraph on the clinical case study of Elijah against the classical reasons for writing a case study (bullet points above). Which of those seems likely to be addressed in this start to the case study? How do I secure the reader's interest in this case study?

An outline answer is given at the end of the chapter.

Writing the case description

One of the things that marks out your case study writing as analytical is the disciplined way in which sections are set out. If the opening of the paper has been to set a scene and capture the reader's interest, the next section exists to describe the case as directly, cleanly and accurately as possible. The case in our instance describes a man and his rehabilitation care, now complicated by delirium. This is the most descriptive part of the paper that you write, although you will need to plan it in a very analytical way. A good way to describe this section is to see it as akin to the way in which a police officer might describe a crime scene. It is important to present all of the relevant facts, those relating to the time and place of the sequence of events. Importantly, though, the police officer does not interpret the scene at this stage; there are no speculative points about needs, motives, relationships or values. The case description describes that which happened, as factually as possible.

I asked Sue (our case study registered nurse) about how that might seem in order to better illustrate what is required. Here is what she said:

> *I think nurses habitually start to interpret experiences and to infer needs and wishes. We want to comfort people. We have become relatively good at second-guessing what is required in different situations. That's not what you want in a case study, though, is it? You should stand back first, describe something, and only then explain your insights afterwards. You don't want to muddy the water, making it harder for the reader to understand how your response fitted with what happened.*

Sue has expressed the key requirement brilliantly. If the reader is to make sense of what the case teaches, then a clear separation has to be made between events and reasoning. We have to set aside our urgent need to interpret and to solve problems. No matter how intuitively we might approach care, there is a need to explain reasoning to others, which requires us to describe a case cleanly in the first instance.

So, in the case study of Elijah, we need a brief account of the chronological events that took place. We need an account of what the patient said or did so that we can appreciate it starkly. We must resist the temptation to interpret it prematurely: 'Of course, Elijah was anxious because ….' We have to decide what slice of time the case study focuses upon. It might be possible to outline the whole of Elijah's time in hospital. Many clinical case studies centre upon a section of time, that which best exemplifies what is of interest in the case study.

Here are three paragraphs of writing about the case that exemplify this very factual focus, this dispassionate report of events and words. They might seem cold to you if you have been used to other reflective forms of writing, but they lend to the case study an objective starting point.

Case study: Elijah, part 3

Elijah spent a total of seven weeks in hospital, first two days on an assessment ward, where despite oxygen therapy his condition deteriorated rapidly, then two weeks on the ICU where he was sedated on an artificial ventilator. After being weaned off the ventilator, he was transferred to a rehabilitation ward where he spent the remaining time (the subject period for this case study). During this rehabilitation period, the patient continued to receive supplemental oxygen using nasal cannula, and he began a programme of physiotherapy to counter his residual dyspnoea, reduce the risks associated with immobility, and begin building his confidence again after what he described as a terrifying event. The physiotherapy regimen consisted of two daily sessions superintended by a therapist, supplemented by two lighter breathing exercise sessions led by the nurse.

During the course of his rehabilitation sessions, Elijah became incrementally more suspicious and then aggressive when the physiotherapist worked with him. The nurses asked him whether he was fearful of what exercising his lungs might do after such an acute illness. They explained that the exercise regime was carefully calibrated to work within his personal limits. On the third day of his rehabilitation exercise regime, Elijah lashed out at the physiotherapist and her assistant, knocking her to the floor. He glared at her from his bed and bellowed, 'What are you doing to me. Who are you anyway? Do they pay you for this. Did they send you to finish the job?!' When the team reviewed this incident and his care leading up to it, they noted that Elijah had started to express severe doubts about the physiotherapist he had assaulted. He had started to rehearse memories that he felt he had from his time in the ICU.

The senior nurse interviewed Elijah and he insisted that he remembered the physiotherapist from before. She had hurt him when he was ill in the ICU (the therapist had no role there, it being a separate red zone isolation facility). Elijah claimed that she had pinched and bruised him. He believed that he had heard her laughing at him. 'They have such low pain thresholds and not an ounce of fight in them', he reported recalling what he believed the therapist had said. The senior nurse reminded Elijah that she had enquired about his ICU experience before, when he had first arrived on the rehabilitation ward. Then he had said that he had no particular memories, just of feeling ill, breathless and frightened. Now he insisted that the physiotherapist had pinched and humiliated him while in the ICU.

What I hope you note in this example is that the case unfolds the problem. In this instance, that centres on patient beliefs and behaviour. Elijah was not obviously agitated, but as time progressed post ICU he became convinced that he had been persecuted there. The nurse checked that there had been no derogatory remarks directed at Elijah in the ICU and that his sedation had been well managed. The nurse established that the physiotherapist had not worked in the ICU. But at this point, no analysis is undertaken. There is no speculation about the effects of sedatives, hypoxia, his state of anxiety when he became ill and was transferred to intensive care. Later, a debate might follow about care standards and respect for the patient. Elijah's memory could be a delirium delusion or it could have a basis in truth. This section, though, is not a place to speculate about Elijah's perceptions of what happened. The purpose is to record what he believed occurred.

Before a problem can be solved, it must be described as clearly and dispassionately as possible. If the patient does not trust those caring for them, collaboration on care becomes difficult. With Elijah, the case description then went on to outline what the nurse then did to address his anxieties. This consisted of four things:

- She introduced the diary entries of the nurses who had cared for him in the ICU. This detailed their names and what they did for him, as well as the routine of his day. The diary entries also included a summary of how he was progressing there.
- She arranged for his lead ICU nurse to speak to him via video call on a mobile phone (Covid-19 protection measures precluded a personal visit from a red zone area). The nurse described how she had looked after him, moving him regularly, watching over him and controlling the machines that breathed for him.
- She described to him how a strange and technical environment, no obvious night or day, medications, and hypoxia can serve to disorientate a patient and evoke vivid memories. Patients might suffer hallucinations or delusions.
- She reviewed Elijah's skin with him in order to ascertain whether there were any marks indicative of recent pinching or other forms of injury. No marks were identified.

The case description detailed that no further physical attacks upon staff followed, but Elijah remained convinced that the same therapist had malevolent intent towards him. The team then elected to assign to Elijah's care a different therapist and continued with their psychological work, piecing together with him the narrative of his illness and care. As no further aggressive outburst followed, he did not receive antipsychotic medication. Elijah eventually left the rehabilitation ward with improved respiratory function and an improving level of mobility, but with entrenched beliefs that the particular therapist had been a threat.

Activity 11.4   Reflection

Why should the case description of your paper be presented very factually, without undue interpretation? What might be problematic if you used it to speculate prematurely?

An outline answer is given at the end of the chapter.

Summarising relevant evidence

So far, the clinical case study has set the scene, creating a focus for the paper, and it has dispassionately described the case. The case has been a patient and his care over a period of time on the rehabilitation ward. We now need to utilise any available evidence that played – or could have played – a role in the case. Not every clinical case study will have a large body of evidence to summarise. Sometimes evidence is sparse, or even non-existent in some areas. But the point of this section is to succinctly summarise evidence that you believe has a bearing on the case in question. The evidence might indicate support for the care measures used or it might raise questions about the care approach. It might be contradictory, with some evidence countering other evidence. The point is that this section sets a wider world of knowledge context to the case in question.

As you have read earlier in Chapter 8, evidence can take different forms, and all of it might be relevant to your chosen clinical case study. You will have to discriminate, though, between what has real purchase for the issue or problem in question and what is much more peripheral and can reasonably be left out. The purpose of this section is not to provide a thorough literature review. It is not an evidence review paper, but an evidence in possible application summary. For that reason, the range of evidence that you might include here may well be rather more circumscribed. It is evidence that has a good fit with the context, with the need or problem identified.

Activity 11.5   Speculation

What evidence do you think might have purchase in a case study such as that of Elijah?

Jot down your answer before reading on.

I hope that you immediately suggested evidence relating to delirium, which causes confusion and anxiety for a patient in or after intensive care. You might have ventured that you would look at evidence relating to beliefs and values, how they are formed and sustained in the context of illness and beyond. Elijah believed that he was being persecuted; irrespective of whether that was factually true, his response to those helping him was sincerely based on the beliefs held. Other evidence of interest includes remedial measures designed to counter delirium in the context of intensive care and its immediate aftermath. Delirium can be tackled using antipsychotic medication, but it might also be addressed using occupational health or psychological measures (Duning et al., 2021).

It might seem unlikely that Elijah was maltreated within the ICU. The claimed perpetrator did not work there, and a survey of the skin revealed no marks or injuries. Elijah was one of several very sick patients in care at the same time and the ICU staff sought to rescue each. However, because we cannot dismiss abuse out of hand, it would be relevant to review any evidence relating to the mistreatment of sedated patients within high-dependency care areas. It would be especially relevant to examine any evidence relating to memory of that heard while under different levels of sedation. While nurses might not like to confront the possibility of maltreatment in care, we should not be complacent.

In this section, you review the nature and extent of the evidence available, whether it seems to relate to the clinical case study in question. Once again, the writing style should be objective and measured. It is not appropriate to jump to conclusions and judge the match of clinical case study care and evidence. Insights and issues are discussed in the next section, so here you are still laying a reasoning trail for the reader, helping them to take stock of what you are considering. Take a look now at some further sample writing from this section of the case study. Here, I am taking stock of the adequacy of evidence available. Is the body of evidence clear and unambiguous? I have not yet applied it to Elijah; I am still reviewing all that might be relevant.

Case study: Elijah, part 4

The above selection of reviewed papers highlights a series of difficulties regarding evidence-based practice and the management of post-ICU delirium. The first is that clinicians vary in their assessment of the significance of delirium. Some 80 per cent of post-ICU patients may suffer a degree of delirium (Weaver et al., 2017), but for the majority it is transitory and relatively easily combatted with reassurance by clinicians. When authors determine that the problem is significant, however, distinctions are made between hypoactive delirium (withdrawal and disengagement) and hyperactive delirium (characterised by anxiety, agitation, and sometimes delusions and hallucinations). The literature varies in its assessment as to which is more important. Hypoactive delirium may undermine rehabilitation as the patient gives up hope, while hyperactive delirium risks self-harm (e.g. the patient ripping out tubes).

Beyond debates regarding the nature of the problem, division then arises as regards best response. Weaver et al. (2017) researched the merits of antipsychotic drugs in terms of the speed with which patients recovered from delirium. They deduced that there was no obvious merit in the use of medications such as haloperidol, which could risk cardiac function in patients that may have been ventilated artificially. Patient counselling or coaching solutions offered a similarly incomplete answer as patients varied in their levels of agitation, as well as how counselling support was then used. There was, however, modest indication that explaining ICU care to patients (continuity follow-up) might benefit patients as they narrated what had happened to them (Haines et al., 2019).

Activity 11.6   Reflection

A question arises as you move towards the next section of your case study, and this centres on the fit of evidence to the circumstances described. In Chapter 8, I described how different types of research might be evaluated. In the clinical case study, however, the focus is on how evidence relates to experience, and vice versa. Each of the following questions might assist you as you weigh up what evidence has to offer:

1.   How coherent is the body of evidence? If research recommends many different and divergent things, the utility value of evidence might currently be low.
2.   Conversely, does the body of evidence suggest that some patient experiences or needs are more important and/or occur more frequently?

3. Does the evidence suggest that one or more interventions are more effective, or else better understood, better received or better evaluated by patients?
4. Does the evidence suggest that something remains ambiguous or contentious? It is here that difficulties might arise for the patient and clinician.
5. Are there any evidence 'black holes' where no one has apparently confronted issues that arose in the case study? Your case study might point to the need for future research.

Think back to a patient that you have nursed in order to judge whether the above evidence in use questions seem valuable. Does this help you to clarify in your mind why sometimes the relevance of evidence is at least as important as its apparent power (e.g. sample size, robust fieldwork methods)?

As this is a personal reflection, no outline answer is offered at the end of the chapter.

Discussing insights and issues

In the penultimate section of your case study, you bring together all of the important points, discussing insights and issues about what the case might teach us. This includes that which was observed from practice and that which is available elsewhere from evidence. It enables you to review what seemed wise, practicable and desirable to the clinician in practice. It considers how the clinicians proceeded, the decisions that they made. In some instances, the nurse might have been unaware of valuable evidence – their practice template was perhaps incomplete. But in other instances, the reasoning may have accommodated factors that research and theorists failed to consider. Sharing insights and issues demonstrates to the reader what you thought significant about the case study and the wider evidence available.

This is often the longest section of the clinical case study, but it still needs to be a disciplined form of writing that shows how you drill down to what is really important. To that end, it is useful to identify and note down the four or perhaps five most important points before you write up the section. My maxim is that it is better to write about fewer things more clearly than it is to range widely, explaining matters ambiguously.

Let us return to the Elijah case study. Here are some points that I speculated as important from the case study:

1. Delirium is not simply a product of altered physiology, medications and treatments. Delirium is experienced individually, and in this case Elijah experiences the insecurities of illness/ICU in racial persecution terms. While there was no objective evidence of mistreatment and the physiotherapist had no contact with the patient in the ICU, Elijah's future care relationship is impacted by his fears and beliefs. It remains debatable whether clinicians can in a short space of time counter deeply held beliefs that may have been informed by past personal experiences. Asking another therapist to work with Elijah was a practical interim step, however.

2. There is a debate about inoculating patients against delirium. The senior nurse used three explanatory measures as a rescue for Elijah, but what if these had been used more strategically to tell his story in the ICU before? This raises questions about how serious delirium is, whether it warrants preventative work.

3. What does Elijah's case tell us about delivering person-centred care in a post-psychological trauma context? Person-centred care starts with the patient's own narrative of need and concern. This case seems to accent that attention needs to focus firmly on Elijah's perceived concerns and needs if he is to partner the nurse in care.

4. Do we really recognise delirium in all of its presentations? Hypoactive delirium (non-engagement, a withdrawn patient rather than agitation, delusions or hallucinations) may in the longer term hamper rehabilitation even more if the patient gives up hope of recovery. Are our patient assessment templates complete?

5. Might other factors have contributed to Elijah's perceptions, fears and aggressive behaviour? For example, there is no mention of him having any contact with family or friends during hospitalisation. Perhaps if there had been, he might have felt less vulnerable. Even where social contact might be possible, it was constrained by Covid-19 protocols, such as wearing personal protective equipment (PPE), which presented a barrier to communication. Could this have exacerbated Elijah's anxieties and fears?

An example of my musing is contained in the following passage.

Case study: Elijah, part 5

In the midst of a pandemic, care resources are stretched to the limit. As patients emerge from ICUs, there is a considerable degree of relief, but recognition too that residual work remains to be done. In the case of Elijah, this certainly centred on physical rehabilitation. There was a clearly reasoned regimen of breathing exercises and graduated mobility training to help Elijah recover his independence. But what also seems certain is that mental health rehabilitation is important as well. Person-centred care (Price, 2022) highlights how the nurse tries to discover the patient's own narrative of injury or illness, their coping and recovery. That seems important in the case of a patient with confusing, frightening and alarming thoughts about what has been happening to them. If the memories are inaccurate, then they still need to be understood. The patient still needs assistance to make sense of their experiences and beliefs so that next step care can be contemplated together. Elijah was not simply another Covid-19 sufferer or ICU survivor; he was a patient trying to make sense of a gap in his recent history, but who still needed physiotherapy now.

Activity 11.7   Reflection

Think back to some other essays that you have written and consider the following maxim also given at the start of this section:

Writing about less, but in rather more detail, is better than writing about a lot superficially.

Do you support the maxim? If you have tried to stretch too far, writing widely before, was that because you imagined that an assessor wanted to know what you knew rather than how you reasoned? If you focused your work more, what gave you the confidence to do that?

As this is a personal reflection, no outline answer is offered at the end of the chapter.

Reaching conclusions

The final section (as in other essays) is made up of your conclusions. You finish the clinical case study by summing up what you deduce from the enquiry. As with other conclusions, it is important to focus this one on what was discussed in the preceding sections of the paper – you should not be raising new issues at this point. The conclusions should relate closely to what you have speculated about in the last section, as well as to the marrying of evidence and experience. You might wonder what constitutes a conclusion, the point where speculation ends. The answer is that a conclusion is where you state your resting position, where you let go of the discussion. Experienced nurses rarely write diatribes in their conclusion. The deductions are measured and nuanced, as befits higher-level critical thinking (see Chapter 3).

Here is a sample paragraph from my conclusion to the Elijah clinical case study. Notice how closely it relates to the speculative points that I raised in the last section of the paper. It is something that I relate to person-centred care and rehabilitation, the introductory context that I started the clinical case study with. A good conclusion brings the reader full circle, back to that which first alerted them to the possible significance of the case study.

Case study: Elijah, part 6

The case study of Elijah offers a salutary lesson about care investment. What seems to mark out the expertise of the nurse is not simply what they say or do, but when they choose to do it. Expert person-centred care is about timely investment. In this instance, the senior nurse uses information to rescue the care of Elijah. She offers diary accounts of his ICU time, a personal greeting from a nurse caring for him there, and an explanation of delirium to help Elijah explain feelings of persecution to himself. She ventures the argument, 'We cannot always trust our memories for these reasons, but here is an account of what was done to help you – you were important to my colleagues.'

(Continued)

(Continued)

This can represent a patch to counter emergent problems. It can, though, when used earlier, represent an inoculation of care. The measures used help to personalise care and assure the patient of proper regard for their needs. What remains problematic, however, is judging when the patient is ready to engage in such a review of events. When Elijah transferred to the rehabilitation ward, he expressed no delusional thoughts. In such circumstances, even against significant time restraints, it might be wise to offer a 'just in case' account anyway. From such an account, new narratives of need and care might begin.

Chapter summary

Clinical case studies offer an excellent opportunity to analyse care over more protracted periods of time, to work with the more familiar care currency (working with a patient and their needs). This seems especially relevant in person-centred care. The clinical case study can serve a number of different professional and academic purposes (e.g. unpicking a problem, relating evidence and experience to each other). Importantly, in this book, case studies can help us to explore how the nurse reasons, revealing the templates that they use to deliver care.

Writing up a clinical case study, though, requires a disciplined writing approach. The case must be chosen with care and with regard to module assessment requirements. Thereafter, the study has to be arranged in a series of strategic sections and utilise a measured, dispassionate form of writing. Each section of the clinical case study builds on the last, and it is important to avoid judging points until issues are discussed and conclusions are reached at the end.

Activities: brief outline answers

Activity 11.1   Critical thinking (page 161)

I would suggest that the clinical case study offers the chance to relate how care was negotiated and planned. This is rarely captured in a reflective practice essay, with its focus on a clinical episode. It is something much more applied than that typically discussed in a theory-based essay. Here, you are able to acknowledge how nurses think in practice, to discover what is sometimes called 'practice wisdom'.

Activity 11.2   Reflection (page 162)

The Covid-19 pandemic presented a tsunami of challenges to nurses, especially those working in areas of high dependency care. Patients such as Elijah kept on arriving and a significant number of them died. I think that Elijah's circumstances test nursing resilience in three major regards.

1.   We are unable to fashion care solutions that seem complete, let alone ideal. We are forced 'back to basics' and there is little opportunity to engage the patient in consulted care. Later, Elijah's perception of past care events will force the nurses to patch care, to reassure in retrospect.

2. Nurses in such tsunami care contexts felt that they had limited treatment resources to fight the Covid-19 infection with. They spent time helping patients to 'hang on' until their immune response improved. It has been over a century since such an impoverished care context was the norm.

3. The sheer volume of patients admitted to hospital forced nurses to cut their cloth, triaging what care could be afforded to each patient. The legacy of this is that nurses often reflect that they had to make terrible decisions.

In such circumstances I wonder if you agree that nursing resilience needs to rest upon an appreciation of what could realistically be delivered, sometimes discrete measures that supported the dignity of patients? Resilience seems to rest too upon just in time care, assessing relative need among a surge of patient admissions. For us to sustain our self-respect in such care contexts we might have to evaluate not the richness or volume of care, but the timing and targeting of care responses. Leaving shift, the nurse might ask, not what did I resolve, but what did I sustain until a patient such as Elijah can partner us more?

Activity 11.3   Critical thinking (page 163)

I venture that this writing promises the analysis of a care problem and it examines care philosophy (person-centred care). I wonder if you felt that the writing attracts you because it raises the question of what happened next. How did they address this problem? In professional writing (for nursing journals), this is called the hook. It draws you into the discussion. A journal reader does not have to read to pass assessments, so the writing has to be professionally compelling.

Activity 11.4   Reflection (page 166)

If you move too quickly to analyse the case, speculating the significance of events, it is then much harder for the reader to distinguish between the events and your interpretations of need. You risk muddying the analysis; were you to do that, an examiner might wonder what you had left out. If you offer only interpretation and no situation, it is difficult to demonstrate your reasoning ability.

Further reading

It is interesting to examine how case studies are used in textbooks.

Kasfiki, E and Kelly, C (2023) *250 cases in clinical medicine*, 6th edition. Edinburgh: Elsevier.

I encourage you to dip into this book to better understand how medical colleagues profile patients as patterns of presenting signs and symptoms. Medicine and nursing have much in common as we must all learn to recognise patterns that might count as problems. The question arises though as to what beyond symptoms and signs we need to understand in order to offer therapeutic support?

Price, B (2022) *Delivering person-centred care in nursing*, 2nd edition. London: Sage/Learning Matters.

My own textbook offers an investigative approach to person-centred care with a clear emphasis on understanding what patients say (their narratives). In this book, the patient comes first, constituting the context for all subsequent discussion of problems and working solutions.

Smith, M (2023) *Clinical cases in augmentative and alternative communication*. Abingdon, Routledge.

The work of the speech therapist is firmly about problem identification, problem solving and rapport building with the client and their family. These case studies explore different techniques used by the therapist to improve the communication of a range of clients and beyond that, their quality of life.

Useful websites

I'd like to invite you to a little exercise which will, I think, help you appreciate the importance of case studies and their relevance to nursing. I offer here a YouTube video from The Michael J Fox Foundation. This offers multiple case study snippet impressions of what it is like to live with Parkinson's Disease. As you view this video ask yourself what case studies can teach you that other sources of information cannot? What is added when you examine experiences side by side? If you were to care for people with Parkinson's disease what key principles would be appropriate to approach them with (your practice template). Here is the weblink:

https://youtu.be/CqEwPqUO1Bw

Case studies afford you opportunities to profile need and to identify key principles that should be born in mind when delivering care. They help articulate how coping articulates with illness and they can illustrate the nature of support requirements too.

Chapter 12 Building and using your portfolio of learning

Chapter aims

After reading this chapter, you will be able to:

- plan the contents of your portfolio so that it addresses academic and professional development goals;
- utilise portfolio elements such as practice templates to illustrate your approach to care;
- build or augment your portfolio in ways that show how your thinking has changed over time.

Introduction

A portfolio of learning might take many forms and the names attached to them may vary as well. They might be called a reflective practice log or diary as well as a portfolio (Telosa-Merlos et al., 2023). Universities differ in the extent to which the portfolio is assessed incrementally over the course and at the end. When portfolios were first developed in nursing, they were often highly structured with pre-set entry pages. Today there seems to be greater latitude for personal choice in the structuring of portfolios and the balance of entries made. Here though I am going to make suggestions that I hope seem coherent to both you and your tutors. As with my commended reflective practice framework (Rolfe et al., 2011), I am going to keep the guidance as clean and as simple as possible.

What is a portfolio?

I define a portfolio as a collated body of information that shows your learning journey during the course. It should indicate something about the state of your learning at point of course completion and signal to others beyond the campus your ability to think, investigate and practise in ways that meet the NMC Code of Conduct (NMC 2018a) requirements and the potential practice roles that you might wish to later pursue. Your portfolio is begun in association with a course of studies, but it is not solely wedded there. Throughout your professional life you will need to evidence your development and skills to employers and to the licensing authorities as you evidence professional update. The contents of your portfolio will grow and change, as you identify different career goals and demonstrate professional updates.

Before we move to some suggested components of your portfolio it seems helpful to use an analogy of how the whole document might work for you professionally. I would encourage you to see your portfolio much as an artist does, displaying their work. To help you with this it is worth visiting a craft website such as www.Etsy.com and reviewing the 'original artwork' offerings there. Searching this term, you will find a collection of artworks (products) that are presented for review and possible purchase (the portfolio offer). Associated with most artworks is a brief description of how it was made (the creative insight). But beyond individual finished products, you should also gain an impression of the focus of the artist's work, what they paint, and the way in which they use materials.

Why have I briefly diverted you to artwork? It is because by the time you conclude your course of studies, I think that you should have amassed enough material in your portfolio for it to look a coherent whole. There should be a selection of products within the portfolio (individual practice reflections, linked by theme, literature reviews, case studies and practice templates) that would enable a reviewer to gain not only a clear sense of what you have studied, but how you think. Just as an artist develops a recognisable style, so a nurse scholar should offer a recognisably professional approach to nursing. If you think about your portfolio in this way, it has a purpose that extends well beyond academic assessments. The portfolio signals something of what you are most committed to in nursing (Cusack and Smith 2020; Samira et al., 2023). In that sense, your portfolio could prove a valuable asset as you pursue particular nursing posts and enter preferred fields of care. No portfolio is ever entirely finished, but it does develop a coherent whole that interested parties can review with you.

Activity 12.1   Critical thinking

Pause now for a moment to think about the significance of the above claims. Your portfolio should include products (finished pieces), there should be something that links them together (themes). What do you think that this means for the incremental selection of things that you add to the portfolio?

My brief answer appears at the end of the chapter.

To help Fatima and Stewart with the organisation of their portfolios I arranged to show them a portfolio from a postgraduate colleague called Emily that I was advising on her aspirations to become a consultant nurse. Clearly, portfolio work at that level was rather more sophisticated than might be expected in an undergraduate course, but nonetheless, Fatima and Stewart agreed that it would be good to see how the work was structured. The portfolio was prepared in Word and was stored online so that Emily could forward samples from the portfolio to employers or other reviewers as appropriate. All of the portfolio components that I now commend below featured in Emily's offering but each is relevant, too, I think for what your portfolio could become. Fatima and Stewart periodically commented on the component parts, and these appear in a series of boxes below.

Reflective practice episodes

Like other students, Emily had started to amass reflective practice episode records within her portfolio. The very earliest ones had been written up using a more complex reflective practice framework which had at first offered reassurance about what to cover, but which over time had proven rather more constraining as regards what she wished to demonstrate. Moving to a simpler framework such as that of Rolfe et al. (2011) allowed her greater latitude to explain and to speculate in ways that seemed inquisitive and entrepreneurial. Emily and I had agreed that consultant nurses often had to innovate and sometimes they needed to challenge conventional wisdom (Wong et al., 2017). For that reason the more flexible reflective framework offered her scope to write imaginatively and critically, something that would be important in more advanced nursing care. La Trobe University (2022) offer an accessible summary of competing reflective practice frameworks (https://latrobe.libguides.com/reflectivepractice/models, accessed 18 May 2023).

Fatima

All of the reflective episodes are arranged under themes and many of them seem to have dated notes added afterwards. I like the theme sections, that makes them more coherent.

(Continued)

(Continued)

Stewart

I suppose that Emily decided themes that seemed most important to her? An obvious way to link reflections on our course would be to modules and their learning outcomes.

One the potential weaknesses of portfolios is that they can contain a scattergun collection of reflective practice episodes. It is then difficult for the reader to deduce what sense you make of them over time. If you don't see a style, a pattern, (my artwork analogy) to the writing then it could seem that you have deduced very little. If you look back to the Tables 3.1 and 3.2, this doesn't signal the highest levels of reasoning.

My own preference is to arrange reflective episodes under themes that make sense to me and fit with my professional goals. Themes such as care negotiation, patient education and psychological support might transcend different modules of study and enable you to include from different placements as you progress through your course. However, if your portfolio is assessed as part of the course structure, then you must comply with any assessment requirements set there. Work might have to be arranged in module sections, but that should not preclude you from adding a theme subtitle to each reflective practice entry made, so that work could be rearranged after qualifying as a nurse if you wished.

Reflective practice entries are a very important part of the portfolio. They offer an insight into your discovery and they can over time show how your reasoning is improving (Johns, 2017). The very selection of your reflective practice episodes tells the reader something about what seems challenging, problematic, exceptional in care to you. Just how many you include is a moot point. Some may be abandoned over time as better ones are added. As a working principle though I would commend fewer well-developed and fuller reflection episodes rather than an army of in-passing, undeveloped reflections.

Activity 12.2   Reflection

Look back over some of the early reflective practice entries you have collected during the course of your studies to date. Do you see any potential themes that might connect them? Themes are important because they help you to conceptualise nursing, to identify patterns of work that might exemplify sound nursing practice. Themes might relate to stages of care, to types of care activity or groups of patients. Have you considered ways (like Emily) to update them, adding notes over the passage of time?

As this is a personal reflection, no answer has been added at the end of the chapter.

Literature reviews

Emily's portfolio offered impressive evidence of analysis within the literature reviews section of her work. She had by that stage completed two systematic reviews of literature following guidelines used by the Cochrane database (see Table 12.1) (Cochrane Organisation, 2023). The first of these related to the strategic use of pharmacological pain relief measures and the second related to the treatment of anxiety, both of which were relevant topics given her interest in working with patients suffering from chronic illness. Other more thematic (less exacting) literature reviews were included, one on psychological coping with illness and one on the role of lay carers in chronic illness. As indicated earlier in this book, it seems unlikely that your course will expect you to complete a systematic review of the literature as per Cochrane, but literature reviews of a more thematic kind are still valuable within your portfolio.

Key Feature	Notes
Carefully focused question, usually about the effectiveness of a treatment or therapy.	Systematic reviews centre of cause-and-effect subject matter, discrete subject matter that can realistically be measured and which is classically examined in randomised clinical control trials.
Precise inclusion and exclusion criteria for studies admitted to the review.	Where data permits the review will, solely feature randomised clinical control trial research. In extremis less rigorous or smaller scale studies might be admitted with clear caveats as regards what will be claimed in the report.
Rigorous and systematic search of the relevant databases, that which is published within academic journals.	Different databases might offer relevant studies for instance those beyond nursing and aimed at other healthcare professionals.
Critical appraisal of the studies	The studies are typically reviewed within reference to positivist paradigm criteria (see Chapter 8) with a particular emphasis upon identifying bias and assessing the scale of the research project in order to judge how transferable results might be.
Data extraction and analysis.	Data from all the studies has to be extracted and compared. In practice, few studies are designed in exactly the same way so data will vary and caution is required when comparing it.
Interpretation and reporting	Most systematic reviews focus upon the claims made relating to a treatment of therapy and address the question, on balance are the claims of efficacy justified. Reviews are rarely as confident when examining reported treatment shortfalls (they may vary study to study).

Table 12.1 Features of a systematic review of the literature (After Cochrane Organisation systematic review principles)

Thematic literature reviews may have been part of assessed coursework (there is no reason why they should not be added to your portfolio) or they may simply represent the end point of a private library exercise.

> **Stewart**
>
> *I like doing literature reviews when a topic 'itches me'. Some of them fall flat, the material just isn't available. I suppose the reviews can go out of date quite quickly too?*

The purpose of literature reviews within a portfolio is three-fold. First, they signal interest within topics that are relevant to your course or career interests. The fact that a literature review might need updating every few years is not damaging in that regard. The second purpose is to indicate your enquiry skills. You have searched a range of databases, research and other evidence literature, but you might also have explored philosophical papers in some areas (see Table 12.2). The Centre of the University of North Carolina offers a simple guide to preparing a theme-based literature review (writingcenter.unc.edu/tips-and-tools/Literature-Reviews). Nurses will need to continue enquiring throughout their careers. The third purpose of including literature reviews within your portfolio is to indicate how you can link reflective practice episodes together. Imagine for instance that you have a series of reflective episodes where patients or families have criticised care. A literature review then on consumerism within healthcare might set expectations in context.

Feature	Notes
Focus upon a clear topic (or address an assignment question set). A question is still asked but it focuses on mapping something rather than measuring cause and effect relationships.	The topic may centre on an illness, or a patient experience, it might focus on a stage of care. It is thematic rather than centred upon a question about the efficacy of a particular treatment.
Clear search parameters are described, the groups of literature admitted into the review, together with your rationale.	Typically research studies are still prioritised where available but they may be designed within the naturalistic or critical theory paradigms (see Chapter 8). Case studies might be included and audit or philosophical papers too.
Clear audit trail of the search through relevant databases.	The reader must appreciate the types of literature that you search and over what span of time it comes. There may be an issue of currency debated if literature is extremely dated.
Critical appraisal of the individual papers.	The critique is likely to vary according to which type of paper is included. Because of this it is much harder to deduce trends, and to anticipate futures and needs resulting from the literature. At best it is likely that the review identifies possible issues for discussion.

Feature	Notes
Information extraction and reporting	The review acknowledges the scope and the completeness of the available literature and it profiles what is available (for instance the balance of research and other information). Typically reminders are added relating to the contexts from which information is taken (this might be very varied). The report identifies themes and issues that are suggested by the literature that which the clinician might attend to in future. Recommendation may be made as regards where future research is required.

Table 12.2   Features of thematic literature reviewing

Activity 12.3   Critical thinking

Imagine for a moment that you have conducted a literature review on a distinctive theme and secured the help of the librarian as regards the choice of best databases to search and search terms to use. But the literature proves thin and perhaps dated. How might you comment upon that within a portfolio?

My suggested answer appears at the end of the chapter.

Case studies

Chapter 11 illustrated what a written case study might look like, so here we turn to their role within your portfolio. The first two components of your portfolio represent what might be called expansion elements. They indicate a great deal about the breadth of your interests and studies. In a nursing course you may have already realised that you are studying dozens of subjects from those that are extremely empirical (e.g. pharmacology, pathology, physiology) to those that are more expressive/aesthetic (e.g. person-centred care, ethics, empathy). In practice though different subject learning has to come together in order to arrive at effective and sensitive care measures. Nurses have to combine different kinds of information in order to arrive at what Rolfe and colleagues (2011) think of as the 'what next?' of reflective practice. Case studies increase the application, the focusing in of your portfolio learning evidence.

Emily chose to include three extended case studies within her portfolio and each of these described the care relationship and strategic planning conducted with the relevant patient and family over a period varying from six to 14 months. Emily and I agreed this plan of action because it seemed important that she could demonstrate the management of a care relationship over an extended period of time.

> **Fatima**
>
> *My case studies have been much shorter than these, but I can see how they combine different sorts of information to explain what we did. I like them because they also explain things about team working, something that can otherwise get lost in a portfolio.*

Activity 12.4 Reflection

Think back now to the analogy of the artist portfolio shared at the start of this chapter. Do you think that case studies can help you draw together different elements of your learning and show something of your own nursing reasoning (that which might be style for the artist)? What might a reviewer learn about your professional interests from the selection of case studies you include?

As this is a reflective activity, no additional answer is added at the end of the chapter.

Practice templates

Throughout this book, reference has been made to the evolution of templates as you make sense of what you have heard, seen and read during the course. Practice templates mean the working notions of what works well, what is appropriate and necessary as you think about different care situations (see Neck et al., 2018 for a cancer nursing exploration of the concept). Practice templates indicate something about what you think patient needs and expectations are and what nursing measures are typically beneficial when delivering care to patients with similar circumstances. A template will also include some points about evidence that are important if care is to be sensitive, effective and efficient.

In a portfolio it is necessary to translate the term template into something that can be read, and Emily and I spent some time agreeing some recurring features within practice templates that she would write. Table 12.3 summarises the recurring features of the templates that were then written up.

Feature	Notes
Brief summary of the context or patient circumstance in which the practice template operates as a start point for negotiated care. For example Emily developed a template relating to taking patient histories.	Practice templates need a context within which to operate; they are not prescriptions for care that applies everywhere and at all times. Remember that the template is a working start point, that which might affirm to patients our grasp of frequently occurring problems and needs, and which might help build rapport quickly.

Feature	Notes
Key principles: the essential things to consider and/or do as part of a strategic approach to care negotiation or patient support. A key principle in Emily's template is that the patient's way of describing a problem, naming it, is always explored and clarified. Without that nurse and patient might operate to different purpose, misunderstanding what is being discussed.	Key principles represent the essence of the nursing approach used, that which is deployed again and again. As I worked with Emily on hers, I emphasised the importance of utility; the principles had to be actionable. If a principle simply expressed a professional ideal, then the practice template is instead a philosophy template, a series of ideals rather than working measures.
Critical evidence: Not all nursing practice is well served by research evidence, but it is important to capture the best of what is available, that which seems relevant, sound and utilisable. Emily started with 14 different pieces of evidence relating to patient history taking and we reduced that to eight pieces, focusing in particular on utility and clarity of guidance afforded.	The practice template doesn't include a literature review, instead each relevant piece of evidence is added as a reference and to that is added a paragraph summarising what the evidence commends. In day-to-day practice nurses struggle to remember copious amounts of evidence so what is included here and used must seem the most robust and the most accessible material.
Caveats: A caveat is a reminder about what might counter a practised approach to the patient in the described context. They are red flags that caution the need to pause and think again. One of Emily's caveats was where patients and relatives offered starkly different accounts of the patient history. In such instances there was a need to proceed with caution as client care objectives might be very different.	You might be surprised that this last part of the practice template doesn't simply say 'actions'. Remember though that the template relates to an approach. Patients (in Emily's portfolio) might require actions that were quite specific to their medical diagnosis. The practice template is not a prescription, it is not a procedure manual, dictating exactly what to do.

Table 12.3 Recurring features of the practice template (portfolio write-up)

Both Fatima and Stewart were impressed with the range and the quality of the practice templates that Emily included within her portfolio. They agreed that these represented a good deal of Emily's expertise, what was particular about the way she approached patient care. Both of the students though had questions to pose about practice templates and their record, which we will now answer in turn.

Stewart

I was wondering how practice templates differ from procedural handbooks such as those published by the Royal Marsden Hospital (Lister et al., 2021)?

For those of you not familiar with the above textbook I would explain that it succinctly combines a wide range of clinical procedures and associated evidence to provide the clearest picture of what the authors commend as sound practice. The procedures covered are all important in cancer-related care but have wider application too.

There is though a difference between practice templates and procedure guides such as the above textbook. The first is that a procedure guide is usually more tightly focused than a template and in many instances, it is more prescriptive. The above textbook was part of the brand identity of cancer care at the Royal Marsden Hospital and it commended excellent standards within such procedures to clinical care elsewhere. Practice templates capture the nursing approach and these focus on rather broader areas of work necessary to establish rapport and build care relationships. If a procedure guide appeals strongly to science as a basis for commended action, then practice templates partner science (evidence), with articulated experience and leave sufficient room for the negotiation of care beyond. In Emily's practice template on patient history taking the account was less about things that must be covered and more about the ordering of enquiry and what needed to be considered.

Fatima

I really like Emily's practice templates, they would encourage me to trust her if she was my nurse. But these collide with standard care pathways, preset nursing care plans don't they?

This is an excellent question. When you write up practice templates you are moving to what you argue you should do in practice rather than what could be done. In Emily's case that was important. She had to portray that she had the confidence, the potential authority to develop nursing practice locally as a consultant nurse. The key principles that she commended, the evidence supporting them could be scrutinised, especially if they suggested a challenge to established local practices. But that, I venture, is the lot of the consultant nurse and to a lesser degree it is the lot of the registered nurse as well. The NMC code of practice (NMC 2018b) makes it clear that the nurse must advocate best practice and protect the well-being of patients. Liaising with others in teams must on occasion involve difference of opinion. Emily might be persuaded to modify her practice template or local practices might change. What is important though would be that the portfolio builder understands why they think as they do and be able to make a considered case for change.

Activity 12.5   Evaluation

Pause now to consider the role that your portfolio might have to play in the clarification of your attitudes, values and beliefs, your reading of evidence to date, that which could create tensions for you in future practice as a registered nurse. If nursing care is not entirely homogenous, why is it important to understand these matters?

My brief answers appear at the end of the chapter.

Discussing your portfolio

Much of this chapter has worked to help you to decide what a portfolio is, how it might serve different purposes and what could be included within it. Before we close the chapter, however, I want to add some suggestions regarding the discussion of your portfolio as it develops over time and when the whole or elements therefore are presented to others as part of your claim to professionalism and expertise.

A professional portfolio benefits from discussion during development (Treloar et al., 2015). In Emily's case, I was the consultant who helped her to think through its development. In your case the person helping is likely to be your personal tutor. While a variety of others might usefully comment on different entries (clinicians and module tutors for example), it is the personal tutor who usually is charged with your development across modules of study. To help your personal tutor give you the best guidance, however, it is important to prepare well. Here are three things to do:

- Before any scheduled meeting, identify the issues that concern you most, the needs that exercise you. Forewarn your personal tutor of the same.
- Send your personal tutor an advance copy of any portfolio entries that help you to summarise the issues of concern. It's unrealistic to ask a personal tutor to speed read entries during the meeting itself.
- Anticipate that your personal tutor will ask you some searching questions about what you supply. In some instances personal tutors commend particular solutions, but often they prompt you to identify solutions of your own.

It's worth remembering that much associated with your development is not a straightforward science matter. Personal tutors differ in how they advise students and this in part results from their own learning experiences and personal skills. So your personal tutor may work with you on your portfolio quite differently to others. In extremis (where your studies or portfolio are going wrong and your progress is in doubt), they will usually be much more directive. In most instances though the guidance suggests what you could do, what might clarify what you wish to explain.

Two other groups of people might review your portfolio with you. The first are course examiners and here the guidance is entirely pragmatic. You should ensure that your portfolio and its entries address the project requirements set. Make sure that the relevant entries are dated and any update notes are added (again dated). Check whether you are required to provide critical summaries of different sections of your portfolio content. Establish whether the assessment requires you to submit your portfolio as a whole or whether illustrative sections of the material are to be submitted. You won't impress your examiner if you send a thick folder of material if only sample reflective episodes are required. Study any assessment requirements added to the assignment. For example, are you required to show how you are relating experience to evidence and back again?

The last group of possible reviewers are those individuals who are selecting nurse candidates for particular posts or project work. In my experience, examples of portfolio work become the more important the higher you progress in your career. A CV or resume might suggest work that you have done, but portfolio entries can illustrate how you have done things. In research, practice development teams, interviewers wish to understand more about how you think and interact. Portfolio entries can help you capture the best of your work, what drives your sense of quality nursing care. Quite often, before a short list of candidates are drawn up for interview, employment panels ask the candidates to submit selective samples of their work. Your portfolio then becomes the resource pool for your application.

If you have not been asked to supply evidence of work/reasoning to date, it is reasonable to make a polite enquiry of whether the supply of sample material might assist the selection panel. If you supply this material before an optional visit to the unit or organisation concerned, this enables them to raise issues from your portfolio submitted during informal discussion/tour of the facilities. It is worth remembering that teams are often quite anxious about the hiring of new colleagues and especially leaders. If they have had the chance to read a sample of how you reason you might reassure or encourage them, something that could make interviewing easier for all concerned.

Chapter summary

The format and content of portfolios may vary widely, dependent upon course requirements but also upon the professional use to which the document is put. Your portfolio might be both a course document (something assessed) but also something that sustains and equips you for the future. There remains though a need to marshal the contents of your portfolio, creating a number of product elements that others can fairly evaluate. Entries such as reflective practice episodes, literature reviews, case studies and practice templates offer an excellent means of representing your experience to date, your reasoning, enquiry and application of ideas to practice.

A portfolio is ideally much more than a document to be completed for assessment purposes. A well-marshalled portfolio can help sustain your studies, giving you avenues to pursue, exploring that which concerns or excites you about nursing. A well-organised portfolio offers a sense of progress, through what Rolfe and others (2011) have described as what, so what and what next?

Activities: brief outline answers

Activity 12.1   Critical thinking (page 177)

The key realisation is that portfolio building should be an incremental but strategic endeavour. It seems unwise to simply collect entries in the happenchance that near the end of your course they might seem to represent something. Sometimes one set of entries will set you off on new related enquiries and that's exactly as it should be if you are to become an independent thinker. Artists think this way too, they build themes of work.

Activity 12.3   Critical thinking (page 181)

Literature reviewing takes a considerable amount of time and effort, so I don't imagine that your portfolio will feature dozens of them. But those that falter are still worth writing up, in terms of identifying where the gaps in the literature are, what has been left unresearched to date and what ambiguities this might pose for policy, practice and your own practice templates. Understanding what is not yet discussed helps us to appreciate why some areas of care remain difficult.

Activity 12.5   Evaluation (page 184)

In my experience attitudes, values and beliefs don't secure the level of discussion that we might hope for in a nursing course. Professional values are fully elucidated (should), but we struggle to examine what it takes to uncover our own attitudes, values and beliefs and perhaps then change them (could). Your portfolio though can help you to uncover personal attitudes, values and beliefs, that which you might discuss with your personal tutor before difficulties arise in practice. While you must practise using the NMC code of practice (NMC 2018b) there still remains scope for discoveries and difficulties. No one starts their course *tabula rasa* without values and beliefs, and, soon, compromises will need to be sought.

Further reading

de Castillo, SLM (2017) *Strategies, techniques and approaches to critical thinking: a clinical reasoning workbook for nurses,* 6th edition. Philadelphia, PA: W.B. Saunders.

This book offers an additional focus on the links between thinking, learning and clinical practice. We share a concern for the pragmatic and skill-based nature of nursing. Much of the text assumes a different healthcare context to that of the UK; but many of the themes remain relevant.

Standing, M (2023) *Clinical judgement and decision making in nursing,* 5th edition. London: Sage/Learning Matters.

Mooi Standing's book on clinical judgement is the logical complement to this one on critical thinking and writing. Mooi elucidates the different ways in which nurses reach clinical decisions, taking into account their experience and patient needs, as well as what I write about as 'utility concerns' (those concerning resources). It's well worth exploring Mooi's text alongside my suggestions regarding practice templates.

Useful websites

I want to end this chapter and the book, with one last visit to a video clip, the sort that I have regularly used to complement the teaching here. I would be very surprised if this simple promotional video for Cleveland Clinic does not move you.

www.youtube.com/watch?v=cDDWvj_q-o8

Empathy: The human connection to patient care.

In the end, I hope that this is where your portfolio takes you, to a more compassionate appreciation of patients and their circumstances. What we offer is not simply treatment, or therapy, or even skill, it is an abiding interest in and respect for their experience and felt needs. I promise you, if your practice templates work here, in such care areas, you are about to embark upon a very fulfilling career and one where you make a profound difference to people's lives.

I hope that this book has seemed a companion to you, with enough 'how to' and 'what about?' to sustain you as you complete your studies. If it has worked, you will feel excited now and, yes, a little more insightful too. My best wishes for your practice.

Glossary

absolute thinking   A low-level form of critical thinking that admits only black or white, right or wrong, and/or good or bad explanations of issues and events.

argument   In formal philosophy terms, an argument is something that states a position and connects to a series of underlying premises that support it. Classically, this involves the inclusion of the word 'because' in the argument. For example, 'Patients are eager collaborators in care planning because they have a vested interest in alleviating personal anxiety and meeting their own goals.' We can begin to test this philosophically when the underpinning premises are then interrogated. For example, do all patients experience anxiety? In nursing course writing and discussion, however, the term 'argument' is more loosely used to refer to a point, that which you claim is relevant, reasonable and pertinent. Such points usually have to be supported by evidence to pass muster at assessment.

case   In academic contexts, the case is a collection of arguments that explains or defends something. For example, a case might state, 'Teaching patients is a key part of nursing practice.' This is supported by a series of arguments: 'Patients need to master self-care.' 'It is more cost-effective for patients to learn self-care.' 'Nurses are interested in supporting patients and their choices and efforts.' In an academic essay, the examiner might set a case for you to discuss, or else require you to formulate a case of your own.

citation   This refers to an acknowledged source of information within your written work. It includes details of the name(s) of the author(s) and the date of publication. Further details, such as the publisher and place of publication, are then added in the reference list at the end of your work.

cognitive intelligence   Ways of reasoning in a rational way, attending to the facts, premises and arguments. Cognitive intelligence relates to the use of logic, unpicking information in a stepwise fashion (see also **emotional intelligence**).

contextual thinking   Thinking about issues, problems and needs with close reference to the context in which they arise. Contextual thinking is nuanced and considered to be a relatively high level of critical thinking.

critical theory   A philosophical and research paradigm that accepts that all knowledge is shaped in some degree by power, and that the rightful role of research is to expose inequality and advance the lot of those who are disadvantaged. Marxist and feminist researchers work in the critical theory paradigm and typically use methods such as action research (collective projects designed to change healthcare).

critical thinking   The process of analysing information and arguments in a methodical way to ascertain what is truthful, reasonable, beneficial and wise. See also my full definition on page 11.

decision-making   That element of critical thinking which signals the nurse's shift in attention or focus, which means that new work has begun. For example, the nurse completing a literature search decides that enough literature has been found. The nurse's effort then moves on to cataloguing the literature. Critical thinking without such activity is not critical at all, representing merely the accumulation of information.

declarative critical thinking   That element of reasoning which relates to our confidence that something is true, proven or viable. For the nurse to proceed with care decisions, for example, certain information has to be declared true, accepted or evident. Without the confidence to assert some facts, particular arguments, critical reasoning and new care cannot proceed.

deductive thinking   The process of testing an idea or theory. This presumes that a theory has been created in the first place. The nurse then tests it out, using research, observations in practice or discussions with professional colleagues. In practice, nurses are continuously deducing what might happen from past experience; they are also inducing ideas, creating theories to explain that which surprised them through care encounters (see also **inductive thinking**).

discourse   An account of what different parties are doing together, which is meant to give substance to the process under way. For example, a discourse on rehabilitation will describe what the nurse and patient do. It will describe their interaction (support, counselling, teaching, guidance, learning). Discourses are sometimes contested and political (e.g. different discourses on the role of the researcher and 'proper science').

emotional intelligence   Ways of reasoning that enable the nurse to quickly identify how events or stances might seem to another, to appreciate how emotions are used to help interpret experience (see also **cognitive intelligence**).

empathy   The ability to identify and have due regard for the experiences and concerns of another. Empathy involves understanding the other person's perspective without necessarily having it determine your own actions. Nurses, for example, have to be empathetic about individual patient needs but independent enough to balance those against the needs of other patients.

empirical   That which can be measured or demonstrated to another. Classically, it refers to acts, documentary accounts or statistics relating to activities. Intentions, values and attitudes only become empirical when they are articulated through action and can be measured in that way. Nursing deals with the empirical world, but it also has to operate within a world of values, beliefs, attitudes and narratives, that which seems emotionally important in the experience of nursing care.

evidence   Information that may support a given nursing argument, stance or plan of action. Traditionally, evidence has been described as a hierarchy, with research evidence at its pinnacle (evidence-based practice). However, other forms of evidence, experience, case studies, audit information and patient satisfaction feedback and statistics are also important evidence to plan care with.

experience   That encountered before and potentially reasoned about to formulate templates for better practice. Where experience is well articulated and critically reviewed, it can contribute to evidence supporting nursing care.

independent thinking   Thinking that involves significant imagination and innovation on the part of the nurse, sometimes described as 'thinking outside the box'. The nurse is sufficiently confident to formulate clear arguments of their own, as well as backing this up with a rationale which suggests that they are able to safely transform nursing practice.

inductive thinking   The process of creating theories or explanations to explain that which has just happened. Induction is important because nurses must constantly make sense of disparate observations and experiences. The diagnosis of a patient need or problem is arrived at incrementally through piecing together observations. This is inductive reasoning (see also **deductive thinking**).

moral justice   A series of ethical arguments about what is right, equitable, fair or just, which is used as the basis of nursing care. While nursing care might advance on the basis of evidence, it might also advance on the basis of moral practice, that which is ethical.

narrative   The storyline of thought that we rehearse to ourselves about what we are doing, why we are doing it, and what purpose it serves. For example, patients develop a narrative to explain what being a patient is, which may or may not fit with the doctor or nurse's expectation of the patient role.

naturalistic (or interpretive)   A philosophical and research paradigm that insists the only way we can authentically understand the world is by studying it in context and trusting respondents to share their experiences and meanings used in the world. The naturalistic paradigm is strongly shaped by social scientists and widely deployed in nursing as researchers explore patient experiences.

paradigm   A widely agreed way of thinking and understanding the world that holds sway over a wide range of thinkers and comes to define how the world should be seen. Thomas Kuhn observed that science moves forward through scientific revolutions, where one paradigm (explanation of the world) is replaced by another. In research, there are currently three paradigms for describing research as an activity: positivist, naturalistic and critical theory.

paraphrase   To express another's arguments within your own paper using your own words. It is critical to cite the source in the text using brackets (author's surname and date of publication). Ensure that you also clearly cite secondary sources drawn upon.

position   Within an essay, the stance that you take on a case made by others. Imagine the case states that all nurses should teach patients self-care. Two obvious stances suggest themselves: either support for or arguments against the case. But a third is also possible: 'Under XYZ circumstances, we cannot readily educate the patient' (perhaps something about the learning ability of the patient).

positivist   A paradigm of research and philosophy that focuses strongly upon the world as a place of facts, traits and dispositions, that which can be explored using the methods of the natural sciences. The emphasis of positivist research is upon carefully controlled design, namely that designed to secure valid and reliable data, as well as that which is open to replication later.

premise   A premise describes that which you accept as true, factual or demonstrable. Arguments are typically built upon premises (that which the nurse accepts as a given) and that which is reinforced by evidence. So, for example, a premise of nursing may be that we help patients to make their own decisions. This is based upon nursing as a profession that helps patients towards their own well-being. Nurses do not direct patients what to do. This sort of premise might support an argument advocating person-centred care.

reflection   The process of thinking in or upon action so as to better understand the event and to ascertain what within it requires the nurse's attention or adjustment. Reflection focuses upon our own and others' actions in order to improve working relationships. See also my full definition on page 28.

seminar   A tutor or group leader discussion where participants return with information and ideas that are designed to shed light on a mutually agreed topic. Seminars require preparation and an active engagement on the part of students, who must share their own discoveries and thinking about that found.

source   Information may come from a primary source (where it was first presented and argued) or a secondary source (where someone else has then commented upon or summarised that original information). Both require citation in an essay.

speculation   The business of supposing or imagining what is happening or required. In nursing, speculation is important – it facilitates more innovative care. The nurse must feel brave enough to speculate about what is wrong and what might help.

template (practice)   A predisposition to reason in a particular way. Nurses develop templates that help them to interpret information smoothly and quickly when dealing with, for example, anxious patients. A rigid template, however, might limit professional development or threaten patient safety. Important principles must be balanced by caveats. What distinguishes clinical reasoning from academic reasoning is the use of templates to address needs and problems in a real-time context, often one where there is an incomplete supply of available information. Template reasoning is pragmatic, weighing needs against resources and using experience to attend to what patients and their relatives, as well as your fellow students, might expect from an encounter. Template reasoning develops over time through paying careful attention to past episodes of care and the critical review of evidence. Templates may be developed around many subjects and enquiries (for example, problem solving) but many in nursing will centre on practice. See Chapter 12 (pp. 182) for commended components of practice templates when written up within portfolios.

transitional thinking   A stage or level of thinking where the individual starts to admit the possibility that a range of factors might shape events or explain what is happening. Transitional thinking suggests that the nurse is starting to see other possibilities, to understand issues in more complex ways.

utility   That which has practical value, which is workable or usable. Not all nursing knowledge has practice utility (i.e. can be deployed at the bedside). However, knowledge may have a professional utility, being of benefit for the ways in which nurses conceive of themselves and their work.

workshop   The process of learning a subject or skill through mutual enquiries and discussion that serve to unpack what is involved. Typically, workshops are used with subjects where there is no perfect or absolutely correct best practice. So, for example, a listening workshop might be convened in association with the support of dying patients. Participants try out explanations of what they are doing while listening; they speculate about what is beneficial or desirable.

References

Aasen, E, Nilsen, H, Dahlborg, E, et al. (2021) From open to locked doors, from dependent to independent: patient narratives of participation in their rehabilitation processes. *Journal of Clinical Nursing*, 30 (–15) 2320–2330.

Adams, L (2016) Learning a new skill is easier said than done. [Online] Available: www. gordontraining.com/free-workplace-articles/learning-a-new-skill-is-easier-said-than-done/ [Accessed 11 November 2023].

Adams, MB, Kaplan, B, Sobko, HJ, Kuziemsky, C, Ravvaz, K and Koppel, R (2015) Learning from colleagues about healthcare IT implementation and optimization: lessons from a medical informatics listserv. *Journal of Medical Systems*, 39(1): 157–62.

Ala-Kokko, T, Erikson, K, Koskenkari, J, et al. (2022) Monitoring of nighttime EEG slow-wave activity during dexmedetomide infusion in patients with hyperactive ICU delirium: an observational pilot study. *Acta Anaesthesiologica Scandinavia*, 66(10): 1211–18.

Allen, D (2022) Wearing religious symbols: what are nurses' rights? *Nursing Standard*, 37(4): 14–16

Ariel, B, Bland, M and Sutherland, A (2021) *Experimental designs.* London: Sage.

Aveyard, H, Preston, N and Farquhar, M (2022) *How to read and critique research: a guide for nursing and healthcare students.* London: Sage.

Aydin Er, R, Sehiralti, M and Akpinar, A (2017) Attributes of a good nurse: the opinions of nursing students. *Nursing Ethics*, 24(2): 238–50.

Baghbani, R, Rakhsham, M, Zarifsanaley, N, et al. (2022) Comparison of the effectiveness of the electronic portfolio and online discussion forum methods in teaching professional belonging and ethical behaviours to nursing students: a randomized controlled trial. *BMC Medical Education*, 22(1): doi: 10.1186/s12909-022-03677-0

Bagnasco, A, Rossi, S, Dasso, N, et al. (2020) A qualitative descriptive enquiry of nursing students' perceptions of international clinical placement experiences. *Nurse Education in Practice*, 43: doi: 10.1016/j.nepr.2020.102705

Bailey, S (2022) *Academic writing for university students.* Abingdon: Routledge.

Barbey, A, Karamn, S, Haier, R (2021) *Intelligence and cognitive neuroscience.* Cambridge: Cambridge University Press.

Barratt, J (2019) Developing clinical reasoning and effective communication skills in advanced practice. *Nursing Standard*, 34(2): 37–44.

Bassot, B (2020) *The reflective journal.* London: Bloomsbury Academic.

Baxter Magolda, MB (1992) *Knowing and reasoning in college: gender-related patterns in students' intellectual development.* San Francisco, CA: Jossey-Bass.

Baylis, D (2015) How to avoid negligence claims. *Practice Nurse,* 45(1): 10–11.

BBC Stories. Fibromyalgia: Living with chronic pain. [Online] Available: https://youtu.be/1CBULIcf9MU [Accessed: 21 September 2023].

Blomberg, K, Lindqvist, O, Werkander Harstäde, C, Söderman, A and Östlund, U (2019) Translating the Patient Dignity Inventory. *International Journal of Palliative Care,* 25(7): 334–43.

Bloom, B (ed) (1956) *Taxonomy of educational objectives: the classification of educational goals.* New York: David McKay.

Bock, A, Idzko-Siekermann, B, Lemos, M, et al. (2020) The sandwich principle: assessing the didactic effect of lectures on "cleft lips and palates". *BMC Medical Education,* 20(310): doi: 10.1186/s12909-020-02209-y

Bolton, G and Delderfield, R (2018) *Reflective practice, writing and professional development,* 5th edition. London: Sage.

Boyd, C (2023) *Reflective practice for nurses.* Oxford: Wiley/Blackwell.

Boyne, J, Chantal, S, Fitzsimmons, D, Hasam, A, et al. (2022) The changing role of patients, and nursing and medical professionals as a result of digitalization of health and heart failure. *Journal of Nursing Management,* 30(8): 3847–52.

Braithwaite, J (2006) Critical thinking, logic and reason: a practical guide for students and academics. [Online] Available: https://www.academia.edu/316239/Critical_Thinking_Logic_and_Reason_A_Practical_Guide_for_Students_and_Aca [Accessed 11 November 2023].

Buchanan, K, Newnham, E, Bayes, S, et al. (2021) Does midwifery-led care demonstrate care ethics? A template analysis. *Nursing Ethics,* 29(1): doi: 10.1177/09697330211008638

Butts, J and Rich, K (2021) *Philosophies and theories for advanced nursing practice,* 4th edition. New York: Jones and Bartlett.

Cadet, M (2018) Iron-deficiency anemia; a clinical case study. *Medsurg Nursing,* 27(2): 108–9 and 120.

Calhoun, EA and Esparza, A (eds) (2017) *Patient navigation: overcoming borders to care.* New York: Springer.

Canadian Arthritis Patient Alliance. Linda Wilhelm's experience of coping with arthritic pain. [Online] Available: https://youtu.be/R45t_vRslCc?feature=shared [Accessed: 21 September 2023].

Carr, VL, Sangiorgi, D, Büscher, M, Junginger, S and Cooper, R (2011) Integrating evidence-based design and experience-based approaches in healthcare service design. *HERD,* 4(4): 12–33.

Casey, M, Cooney, A, O'Connell, R, Hegarty, J-M, Brady, A-M, O'Reilly, P, et al. (2017) Nurses', midwives' and key stakeholders' experiences and perceptions on requests to demonstrate the maintenance of professional competence. *Journal of Advanced Nursing,* 73(3): 653–64.

Chatfield, T (2022) *Critical thinking: your essential guide,* 2nd edition. London: Sage.

Chirillo, M, Silverthorn, D and Vijovic, P (2021) Core concepts in physiology: teaching homeostasis through pattern recognition. *Advances in Physiology Education*, 45(4): 812–29.

Clemett, V and Raleigh, M (2021) The validity and reliability of clinical judgement and decision making skills assessment in nursing: a systematic literature review. *Nurse Education Today*, 102(July): 104885.

Close, E, Wilmott, L and White, B (2021) Regulating voluntary assisted dying practice: a policy analysis from Victoria, Australia. *Health Policy*, 125(11): doi: 10.1016/j.healthpol.2021.09.003

Cochrane Organisation (2023) Cochrane handbook for systematic reviews of interventions version 6.4 [Online] Available: https://training.cochrane.org/handbook/current [accessed 10 November 2023].

Compton, RM, Owilli, AO, Norlin, EE and Hubbard Murdoch, NL (2020) Does problem-based learning in nursing education empower learning? *Nurse Education in Practice*, 44. doi: 10.1016/nepr.2020.102752

Corcoran, L and Cook, K (2023) The philosophy of Hans Georg Gadamer: an example of the complicated relationship between philosophy and nursing practice. *Nursing Inquiry*, 30(1): doi: 10.1111/nin.12509

Creswell, JW and Creswell, JD (2018) *Research design: qualitative, quantitative, and mixed methods approaches*, 5th edition. London: Sage.

Cui, J, Li, F and Shi, Z-L (2019) Origin and evolution of pathogenic coronaviruses. *Nature Reviews Microbiology*, 17(3): 181–92.

Cusack, L and Smith, M (2020) *Portfolios for nursing, midwifery and other health professions*. Edinburgh: Elsevier.

De Bruin, S, Buist, Y, Hassink, J and Vaandrager, L (2021) 'I want to make myself useful': the value of nature-based adult day services in urban areas for people with dementia and their family carers. *Ageing and Society*, 41(3): 582–604.

de Castillo, SLM (2017) *Strategies, techniques and approaches to critical thinking: a clinical reasoning workbook for nurses*, 6th edition. Philadelphia, PA: WB Saunders.

Dickey, l and Botzer, M (2021) *Case studies in clinical practice with trans and gender non-binary clients*. London: Jessica Kingsley.

Dolan, S, Nowell, L and McCaffrey, G (2022) Pragmatism as a philosophical foundation to integrate education, practice, research and policy across the nursing profession. *Journal of Advanced Nursing*, 78(10): e118–e129.

Dubiel, C, Hiebert, B, Stammers, A, et al. (2022) Delirium definition influences prediction of functional survival of patients one-year postcardiac surgery. *Journal of thoracic and Cardiovascular Surgery*, 163(2): 725–37.

Duning, T, Liting-Reuke, K, Beckhuis, M, et al. (2021) Postoperative delirium-treatment and prevention. *Current Opinion in anaesthesiology*, 34(1): 27–39.

Edwards, S (2017) Reflecting differently. New dimensions: reflection-before-action and reflection-beyond-action. *International Practice Development Journal*, 7(1): 1–14.

Ellis, P (2019) *Evidence-based practice in nursing*, 4th edition. London: Sage/Learning Matters.

Ellis, P, Standing, M and Roberts, S (2020) *Patient assessment and care planning in nursing*, 3rd edition. London, Sage.

Esterhuizen, P (2023) *Reflective practice in nursing*, 5th edition. London: Sage/Learning Matters.

Feeney, Á and Everett, S (2020) *Understanding supervision and assessment in nursing*. London: Sage.

Feistauer, D and Richter, T (2017) How reliable are students' evaluations of teaching quality? A variance components approach. *Assessment and Evaluation in Higher Education*, 42(8): 1263–80.

Fisher, M, McKechnie, D and Pryor, J (2020) Conducting a critical review of the research literature. *Journal of the Australasian Rehabilitation Association*, 23(1): 20–29.

Fjortoft, A, Oksholm, T, Delmar, C, et al. (2020) Home-care nurses' distinctive work: a discourse analysis of what takes precedence in changing healthcare services. *Nursing Inquiry*, 28: 28e12375.

Flyverbom, M (2019) *The digital prism: transparency and managed visibilities in a datafied world*. Cambridge: Cambridge University Press.

Fox, M (Michael J Fox Foundation) Living with Parkinson's disease. [Online] Available: https://youtu.be/CqEwPqUO1Bw [Accessed: 21 September 2023].

Fox, P Adult learning theory: Knowles' 6 assumptions of adult learners. [Online] Available: https://youtu.be/SArAggTULLU [Accessed: 21 September 2023].

Gobet, F (2005) Chunking models of expertise: implications for education. *Applied Cognitive Psychology*, 19(2): 183–204.

Gobet, F and Chassy, P (2008) Towards an alternative to Benner's theory of expert intuition in nursing: a discussion paper. *International Journal of Nursing Studies*, 45(1): 129–39.

Gold, AL, Shechner, T, Farber, MJ, Spiro, CN, Leibenluft, E, Pine, DS, et al. (2016) Amygdala-cortical connectivity: associations with anxiety, development, and threat. *Depression and Anxiety*, 33(10): 917–26.

Grant, A, McKimm, J and Murphy, F (2017) *Developing reflective practice: a guide for medical students, doctors and teachers*. Chichester: Wiley-Blackwell.

Greetham, B (2022) *How to write better essays*, 5th edition. London: Bloomsbury Academic.

Grey, D and Osborne, C (2020) Perceptions and principles of personal tutoring. *Journal of Further and Higher Education*, 44(93): 285–300.

Gross, J, Lakey, B, Lucas, J, et al. (2015) Forecasting the student-professor matches that result in unusually effective teaching. *British Journal of Educational Psychology*, 85(1): 19–33.

Gurley, K, Edlow, J, Burstein, J, et al. (2021) Errors in decision making in emergency medicine: the case of the landscaper's back and root cause analysis. *Annals of Emergency Medicine*, 77(2): 203–10.

Hagg-Martnell, A, Hull, H and Kiessing, A (2016) Community of practice and student interaction at an acute medical ward: an ethnographic study. *Medical Teacher*, 38(8): 793–802.

Haines, KJ, Savin, CM, Hibbert, E, Boehm, LM, Aparanji, K, Bakhru, RN, et al. (2019) Key mechanisms by which post-ICU activities can improve in-ICU care: results of the international THRIVE collaboratives. *Intensive Care Medicine*, 45(7): 939–47.

Hamm, B (2021) Ethical practice in emergency psychiatry: common dilemmas and virtue-informed navigation. *The Psychiatric Clinics of North America*, 44(4): 627–38.

Harrison, G and McManus, K (2017) Clinical reasoning in the assessment and intervention planning for writing disorder. *Canadian Journal of School Psychology*, 32(1): 73–87.

Hashemiparast, M, Negarandeh, R and Theofanidis, D (2019) Exploring the barriers of utilizing theoretical knowledge in clinical settings: a qualitative study. *International Journal of Nursing Sciences*, 6(4): 399–405.

Hedesan, J and Tendler, J (2017) *An analysis of Thomas Kuhn's The Structure of Scientific Revolutions*. London: Macat Library/Routledge.

Hediye, U and Seher, Y (2022) The theory-practice gap in nursing education during the pandemic period from the perspective of stakeholders: a qualitative study. *Clinical and Experimental Health Sciences*, 12(2): 499–506.

Heinrich, P (2018) *When role play comes alive: a theory and practice.* London: Palgrave Macmillan.

Hernandez-Acevedo, B, Lundy, T, Clifton, M and Mathew, M (2022) Active learning strategies to enhance student success. *Journal of Nursing Education*, 61(3): 167.

Honeycutt, K and Miller, D (2021) Learner metacognitive insights from writing professional clinical practicum reflections: an instrumental case-study of a university-based MLS program. *Journal of Allied Heath*, 50(1): 57–73.

Huber, E, Kleinknecht-Dolf, M, Kugler, C and Spirig, R (2021) Patient-related complexity of nursing care in acute care hospitals – an updated concept. *Scandinavian Journal of Caring Sciences*, 35: 178–95.

Jack, K and Levett-Jones, T (2022) A model of empathetic reflection based on the philosophy of Edith Stein: a discussion paper. *Nurse Education in Practice*, 63: 103389.

Jakobsen, L and Maehre, K (2023) Can a structured model of ethical reflection be used to teach ethics to nursing students? An approach to teaching nursing students a tool for systematic ethical reflection. *Nursing Open*, 10(2): 721–29.

Jankowski, T (2016) *Expert searching in the Google age.* New York: Rowman and Littlefield.

Jen (2021) How to take effective lecture notes – my best note taking tips and tools. Prep with Jen. [Online] Available: *YouTube.* https://youtu.be/hl-2TxkEwn0 [Accessed 11 November 2023].

Johns, C (2017) *Being a reflective practitioner*, 5th edition. Chichester: John Wiley.

Jolly, J (2020) *Introducing research and evidence-based practice for nursing and healthcare professionals.* Abingdon: Routledge.

Jones, A (2018) *Questioning: pose, pause, pounce, bounce.* Herts and Bucks Teaching School Alliance. [Online] Available: https://hertsandbuckstsablog.wordpress.com/2018/05/17/questioning-pose-pause-pounce-bounce/ [Accessed 11 November 2023].

JuHee, L, Young, J and Minjeong, S (2016) Registered nurses' clinical reasoning skills and reasoning process: a think aloud study. *Nurse Education Today*, 46(November): 75–80.

Kaihlanen, AM, Haavisto, E, Strandell-Laine, C and Salminen, L (2018) Facilitating the transition from a nursing student to a registered nurse in the final clinical practicum: a scoping literature review. *Scandinavian Journal of Caring Sciences*, 32(2): 466–77.

Kasfiki, E and Kelly, C (2023) *250 Cases in Clinical Medicine*, 6th edition. Edinburgh: Elsevier.

Kayambankadzanya, R, Schell, C, Warnberg, M and Mollazadegan, T (2022) Towards definitions of critical illness and critical care using concept analysis. *BMJ Open*, 12(9): e060972.

Kirkpatrick, A (2020) Interpersonal competence development through online palliative care education and virtual interprofessional simulation. *Journal of Pain and Symptom Management*, 60(1): 277–86.

Kirschner, P and Hendrick, C (2020) *How learning happens: seminal works in educational psychology and what they mean for practice.* Abingdon: Routledge.

Ko, LN, Rana, J and Burgin, S (2019) Teaching & learning tips 5: making lectures more 'active'. *International Journal of Dermatology*, 57(3): 351–4.

Koivisto, J-M, Multisilta, J, Niemi, H, Katajisto, J and Eriksson, E (2016) Learning by playing: a cross-sectional descriptive study of nursing students' experiences of learning clinical reasoning. *Nurse Education Today*, 45: 22–8.

Kroemeke, A (2016) Changes in well being after myocardial infarction: does coping matter? *Quality of Life Research*, 25(10): 2593–601.

Kuhn, TS (2012) *The structure of scientific revolutions*, 50th anniversary edition. Chicago, IL: University of Chicago Press.

Lee, JJ, Clarke, CL and Carson, MN (2018) Nursing students' learning dynamics and influencing factors in clinical contexts. *Nurse Education in Practice*, 29: 103–9.

Lee, K-C, Yu, C-C, Hsieh, P-L, Li, C-C and Chao, Y-FC (2018) Situated teaching improves empathy learning of the students in a BSN program: a quasi-experimental study. *Nurse Education Today*, 64: 138–43.

Lee, M, Jones, C, White, P et al. (2023) Preparing health professional students for interprofessional practice related to neurodevelopmental disabilities: a pilot program. *Journal of Interprofessional Care*, 37(2): doi: 10.1080/13561820.2022.2047906

Linsley, P and Kane, R (2022) *Evidence-Based Practice for Nurses and Healthcare Professionals*, 5th edition. London: Sage.

Lister, S, Herfland, J et al. (2021) *The Royal Marsden Manual of Clinical Nursing Procedures, Student Edition*, 10th edition. Chichester: Wiley/Blackwell.

Magnusson, J and Zackariasson, M (2018) Student independence in undergraduate projects: different understandings in different academic contexts. *Journal of Further and Higher Education*, 43(10): 1404–19.

Mahotra, A and Kumar, A (2021) Breaking the Covid-19 barriers to health professional training with online simulation. *Simulation in Healthcare*, 16(1): 80–81.

Maio, G (2016) *The psychology of human values.* Abingdon: Routledge.

Marx, EW and Padmanabhan, P (2020) *Healthcare digital transformation: how consumerism, technology and pandemic are accelerating the future.* London: Routledge.

Mason, CH (2005) Addressing complex health issues: developing contextual knowing through sequenced writing and presentations. *International Journal of Nursing Education Scholarship*, 2(1): doi: 10.2202/1548-923x.1149

Matthews, J (2020) How to write an awesome paragraph: step by step. Amazon (independently published).

Mbutho, N and Hutchings, C (2021) the complex concept of plagiarism: undergraduate and postgraduate student perspectives. *Perspectives in Education*, 39(2): 67–82.

McBee, E, Ratcliffe, T, Schuwirth, L, O'Neill, D, Meyer, H, Madden, SJ, et al. (2018) Context and clinical reasoning: understanding the medical student perspective. *Perspectives on Medical Education*, 7(4): 256–63.

McCarthy, B, McCarthy, J, Trace, A and Grace, P (2018) Addressing ethical concerns arising in nursing and midwifery students' reflective assignments. *Nursing Ethics*, 25(6): 773–85.

McLaughlin Library. What is critical reflection? Introducing the 'what, so what and now what model'. [Online] Available: https://youtu.be/vGyjF9Ngd8Y [Accessed: 21 September 2023].

McPherson, F (2020) *Effective notetaking*, 3rd edition. Wellington: Wayz Press.

Medical Health TV. Interviewing a patient with Parkinson's Disease. [Online] Available: https://youtu.be/AkqFqAksxOU [Accessed: 05 February 2023].

Merisier, S, Larue, C and Boyer, L (2018) How does questioning influence nursing students' clinical reasoning in problem-based learning? A scoping review. *Nurse Education Today*, 65: 108–15.

Michalowsky, B, Henning, E, Radke, A, et al. (2020) Attitudes towards advanced nursing roles in primary dementia care: results of an observational study in Germany. *Journal of Advanced Nursing*, 77(4): 1800–12.

Mitrea, N, Gerzevitz, D, Mathe, T, et al. (2022) Palliative care masterclass for nurses in Central Eastern Europe: an international collaboration. *Journal of Hospice and Palliative Nursing*, 24(3): E83–E92.

Morgan, R (2019) Using seminars as a teaching method in undergraduate nurse education. *British Journal of Nursing*, 28(6): 374–6.

MTa Learning (2021) Use the 'What? So what? Now what?' model: a great example of reflective questioning. [Online] Available: www.experientiallearning.org/blog/what-so-what-now-what-reflection-model-and-reflection-questions/ [Accessed 11 November 2023].

Nagel, J, Chevanon, M, Binder, L, et al. (2021) How family history of premature myocardial infarction affects patients at cardiovascular risk. *Health Psychology*, 40(11): 754–66.

Nak, G, Hendy, R and Harker, N (2018) Developing best practice cancer treatment scanning templates. *Cancer Nursing Practice*, doi: 10.7748/cnp2018.e1500.

Nakayoshi, Y, Takase, M, Niitami, M, et al. (2021) Exploring factors that motivate nursing students to engage in skills practice in a laboratory setting: a descriptive qualitative design. *International Journal of Nursing Sciences*, 8(1): 79–86.

Neff, I (2019) Vital and enchanted: Jane Bennett and new materialism for nursing philosophy and practice. *Nursing Philosophy*, 21(2): e12273.

Nelson-Brantley, HV, David Bailey, K, Batcheller, J, Bernard, N, Caramanica, L and Snow, F (2019) Grassroots to global: the future of nursing leadership. *JONA The Journal of Nursing Administration*, 49(3): 118–20.

Nursing and Midwifery Council (NMC) (2018a) *The code: professional standards of practice and behaviour for nurses, midwives and nursing associates.* [Online] Available: www.nmc.org.uk/globalassets/sitedocuments/nmc-publications/nmc-code.pdf [Accessed 11 November 2023].

Nursing and Midwifery Council (NMC) (2018b) *Future nurse: standards of proficiency for registered nurses.* [Online] Available: www.nmc.org.uk/globalassets/sitedocuments/education-standards/future-nurse-proficiencies.pdf [Accessed 11 November 2023].

Nursing and Midwifery Council (NMC) (2019) *Revalidation.* [Online] Available: www.nmc.org.uk/globalassets/sitedocuments/revalidation/how-to-revalidate-booklet.pdf [Accessed 11 November 2023].

O'Sullivan, B, Hickson H, Kippen, R and Wallace, G (2021) Exploring attributes of high-quality clinical supervision in general practice through interviews with peer recognized GP supervisors. *Medical Education*, 21: 1–10.

Outlaw, K and Rushing, D (2018) Increasing empathy in mental health nursing using simulation and reflective journaling. *Journal of Nursing Education*, 52(12): doi: 10.3928/01484834-20181119-13.

Peltzer, S, Kostler, U, Müller, H, et al. (2022) The psychological consequences of living with coronary heart disease: are patients' psychological needs served? A mixed-method study in Germany. *Health Expectations*, 25(6): doi: 10.1111/hex.13467.

Pope, C and Mays, N (2020) *Qualitative research in healthcare*, 4th edition. Chichester, Wiley/Blackwell.

Presti, CR (2019) Peer learning and role-play to enhance critical thinking. *Nurse Educator*, 44(1): 33.

Price, B (1990) *Body image: nursing concepts and care.* London: Prentice Hall.

Price, B (2003) Academic voices and the challenges of tutoring. *Nurse Education Today*, 23(8): 628–37.

Price, B (2014) Avoiding plagiarism: guidance for nursing students. *Nursing Standard*, 28(26): 45–51.

Price, B (2016) Enabling patients to manage altered body image. *Nursing Standard*, 31(16–18): 60–71.

Price, B (2017) How to write a reflective practice case study. *Primary Health Care,* 27(9): 35–42.

Price, B (2022) *Delivering person-centred care in nursing,* 2nd edition. London: Sage/Learning Matters.

Roberts, M (2015) *Critical thinking and writing for mental health nursing students.* London: Sage/Learning Matters.

Rolfe, G, Jasper, M and Freshwater, D (2011) *Critical reflection in practice: generating knowledge for care,* 2nd edition. London: Palgrave Macmillan.

Rosina, R, McMaster, R, Cleary, E, et al. (2022) Preparing for the real world: clinical facilitators and nursing student clinical placements. *Issues in Mental Health Nursing,* 43(3): 386–9.

Ryan, CL and McAllister, MM (2020) Professional development in clinical teaching: an action research study. *Nurse Education Today,* 85: 104306. doi: 10.1016/j.nedt.2019.104306

Sala, G and Gobet, F (2017) Experts' memory superiority for domain-specific random material generalizes across fields of expertise: a meta-analysis. *Memory & Cognition,* 45: 183–93.

Salifu, DA, Gross, J, Salifu, MA and Ninnoni, JPK (2019) Experiences and perceptions of the theory-practice gap in nursing in a resource-constrained setting: a qualitative description study. *Nursing Open,* 6(1): 72–83.

Samira, M, Tang, L, Chong Mei, C, et al. (2023) The effects of professional portfolio learning on nursing students' professional self concepts in geriatric adult internships: a quasi-experimental design. *BMC Medical Education,* 23(1): 1–13.

Schön, DA (1987) *Educating the reflective practitioner: toward a new design for teaching and learning in the professions.* San Francisco, CA: Jossey-Bass.

Secunda, K, Wirpsa, J, Neely, K, et al. (2020) Use and meaning of 'goals of care' in the healthcare literature: a systematic review and qualitative discourse analysis. *Journal of General Internal Medicine,* 35(5): 1559–66.

Shackleton-Jones, M (2023) *How people learn: a new model of learning and cognition to improve performance and education,* 2nd edition. London: Kogan-Page.

Shakeel, AK and Bhatti, R (2018) Semantic web and ontology-based application for digital libraries: an investigation from LIS professionals in Pakistan. *The Electronic Library,* 36(5): 826–41.

Singh, M (2021) Inroad of digital technology in education: age of digital classroom. *Higher Education for the Future,* 8(1): doi: 10.1177/2347631120980272

Skela-Savič, B, Hvalič-Touzery, S and Pesjak, K (2017) Professional values and competencies as explanatory factors for the use of evidence-based practice in nursing. *Journal of Advanced Nursing,* 73(8): 1910–23.

Skirbekk, H, Hem, M and Nortvedt, P (2018) Prioritizing patient care: the different views of clinicians and managers. *Nursing Ethics,* 25(6): doi: 10.1177/0969733016664977.

Smith, M (2023) *Clinical cases in augmentative and alternative communication.* Abingdon: Routledge.

Smith, PK, Cowie, H and Blades, M (2015) *Understanding children's development*, 6th edition. Chichester: Wiley-Blackwell.

Sokol, D (2018) *Tough choices: stories from the front line of medical ethics*. London: Book Guild.

Standing, M (2023) *Clinical judgement and decision making in nursing*, 5th edition. London: Sage/Learning Matters.

Stein-Parbury, J (2021) *Patient and person: interpersonal skills in nursing*, 7th edition. Edinburgh: Elsevier.

Strawson, H, Habeshaw, S, Habeshaw, T and Gibbs, G (2021) *53 interesting things to do in your seminars and tutorials: tips and strategies for the running of really effective small groups*. London: Routledge.

Struggling with Pain. [Online] Available: https://youtu.be/FPpu7dXJFRI?feature=shared [Accessed: 21 September 2023].

Supady, A, Curtis, R, Brown, C, et al. (2021) Ethical obligations for supporting healthcare workers during the Covid-19 pandemic. *European Respiratory Journal*, 57(2): 1459–61.

Telosa-Merlos, D, Morena-Poyato, A, Gonzalez-Paulau, F, et al. (2023) Exploring the therapeutic relationship through the reflective practice of nurses in acute mental health units: a qualitative study. *Journal of Clinical Nursing*, 32(1–2): 253–63.

Tiffin, P and Paton, L (2020) When I say … emotional intelligence. *Medical Education*, 54: 598–9.

Torres, R and Nyaga, D (2021) *Critical research methodologies*. Chicago: Haymarket Books.

Tracy, S (2019) *Qualitative research methods: collecting evidence, crafting analysis, communicating impact*, 2nd edition. Chichester: Wiley/Blackwell.

Treloar, A, Stone, T, McMillan, M and Flakus, K (2015) A narrative in search of a methodology. *Perspectives in Psychiatric Care*, doi: 10.1111/ppc.12081

Trocky, NM and Buckley, KM (2016) Evaluating the impact of wikis on student learning: an integrative review. *Journal of Professional Nursing*, 32(5): 364–76.

University of North Carolina (Writing Centre) How to write a literature review. https://writingcenter.unc.edu/tips-and-tools/literature-reviews/ (accessed 21 September 2023).

US Pain Foundation Incorporated. Marqus V's chronic pain story. [Online] Available: https://youtu.be/VG-T4pPIWA8 [Accessed: 21 September 2023].

Van Humbeeck, L, Mulfait, S, Van Biesen, W, et al. (2020) Value discrepancies between nurses and patients: a survey study. *Nursing Ethics*, 27(4): 1044–55.

Wallace, M and Wray, A (2021) *Critical reading and writing for postgraduates*, (Student Success), 4th edition. London: Sage.

Walsh, D and Dixon, J (2021) *The nurse mentor's handbook: supervising and assessing students in clinical practice*, 3rd edition. Maidenhead: Open University Press.

Weaver, CB, Kane-Gill, SL, Gunn, SR, Levent, K and Smithburger, PL (2017) A retrospective analysis of the effectiveness of antipsychotics in the treatment of ICU delirium. *Journal of Critical Care*, 41: 234–9.

Whitman, JC, Zhao, J and Todd, RM (2017) Alternation between different types of evidence attenuates judgments of severity. *PLoS ONE*, 12(7): e0180585.

WikiHow. How to reason: 9 steps (with pictures) (2019). [Online] www.wikiHow.com/Reason [Accessed 11 November 2023].

Wilson, B, Woollands, A and Barrett, D (2019) *Care planning: a guide for nurses*, 3rd edition. London: Routledge.

Wolf, A (2018) The impact of web-based video lectures on learning in nursing education: an integrating review. *Nursing Education Perspectives*, 39(6): E16–E20.

Wolff, M, Wagner, MJ, Poznanski, S, Schiller, J and Santen, S (2015) Not another boring lecture: engaging learners with active learning techniques. *Journal of Emergency Medicine*, 48(1): 85–93.

Wong, F (2018) A phenomenological research study: perspectives of student learning through small group work between undergraduate nursing students and educators. *Nurse Education Today*, 68(September): 153–8.

Wong, F, Lau, A, Ng, R, et al. (2017) An exploratory study on exemplary practice of nurse consultants. *Journal of Nursing Scholarship*, 49(5): 548–56.

Young, K, Godbold, R and Wood, P (2019) Nurses' experiences of learning to care in practice environments: a qualitative study. *Nurse Education in Practice*, 38: 132–7.

Zafeer, H, Yangping, L, and Maqbool, S (2023) An approach to progress testing outcomes: international graduate students' engagement in reflective practice and reflective journal writing during pandemic. *Sustainability*, 15(3): doi: 10.3390/su/5031898

Index

Note: References in italics are to figures, those in bold to tables; 'g' refers to the Glossary.